A Beginner's Guide to
Lifting Depression

Leslie O. Simpson, Ph.D.
Research Biologist
Hemorheologist

Nancy Blake, BA, CQSW
UKCP-Accredited Neurolinguistic
Psychotherapist for over twenty years

Note: Your doctor hasn't been taught hemorheology and your therapist hasn't been taught NLP, so you won't find this information anywhere else!

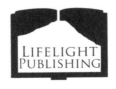

LIFELIGHT
PUBLISHING

Published by Lifelight Publishing 2015

www.lifelightpublishing.com

Cover photo and design by Grainger Graphics

Copyright © Leslie O. Simpson & Nancy Blake 2015

www.nancyblakealternatives.com

British Library Cataloguing in Publication Data. A catalogue record for this book is available from the British Library.

ISBN: 0-9571817-6-0
ISBN-13: 978-0-9571817-6-2

10 9 8 7 6 5 4 3 2 1

A Beginner's Guide to Lifting Depression

THANK YOU

Les would want to thank both his family who are caring for him, and the hemorhologists who have been his inspiration.

Nancy would like to thank the usual suspects…

Sue Walsh for ongoing support and encouragement.

Tony Blake for moral support and his generosity with proofreading and editing.

Phil Grainger for his dedication and frightening competence, as well as willingness to stay on the phone for three hours while I dither about shades of blue.

Sue Grainger – my model for just getting on with the writing – and - immense gratitude for the cover photo….isn't it amazing!

And to Les…..without him none of this would have happened…..

CONTENTS

FOREWORD

Almost any of us would admit to feeling depressed at times, and most of us would be able to pinpoint a reason. But we know that depression can range from a few days of feeling low to weeks, months or years of a devastating sense of despair, guilt, hopelessness and apathy, often without any cause that makes sense to us. This may alternate with periods of relative emotional wellbeing; it may occur only once, or a few times during our life, or may be long-standing.

Les Simpson and Nancy Blake have collaborated on this book for the purpose of providing information about our complementary suggestions for helping yourself, or anyone you may be involved with or caring for, who is suffering from depression.

We write with the proviso that our information does not in any way offer a substitute for the medical advice of your doctor or psychiatrist. Depression is an illness with a very high morbidity and mortality rate as a result of suicide, attempted or successful. Its dangers should not be underestimated. If you, or someone close to you is thinking of suicide, seek help, immediately. It is a myth that people who talk about suicide don't do it—many who talk about it are doing so because they want someone to give them help to prevent it, so see that that help is obtained. You might feel embarrassed if you have taken a threat of suicide too seriously, but you could suffer a lifetime of regret if you hadn't taken it seriously enough.

If you are reading this book, you are looking for help, you are looking for some answers. We very much hope that what we offer will give you, if not answers, at least some ideas that you can try out that may be helpful.

We should add that if you are currently taking prescribed medication for depression, and as a result of trying out our suggestions, you begin to feel better, be sure only to undertake reduction of medication under the supervision of your doctor.

INTRODUCTION

Les Simpson, on the basis of a thirty-year career in hemorheology[1] research, presents a very sound case for the central role of blood flow in depression, and for the effectiveness of life-style changes and easily available supplements which can address this issue.

Nancy's view, on the basis of a thirty-year career as a psychotherapist, is that most depression is 'about something' in the person's current circumstances or past life, and that these issues need to be addressed. She finds the deceptively simple techniques offered by NLP can often cut through the thought patterns of depression more quickly and effectively than traditional forms of therapy, or CBT. She also welcomes the information that an individual's emotional state can be radically improved through the measures that Les recommends.

Les and Nancy both believe in a virtuous circle—improved blood flow will improve mood, and that in turn may give the person the courage and confidence to tackle any issues in their lives which may need to be dealt with in order to make a permanent change.

---

[1] Hemorheology is the study of the physical properties of blood. Unlike haemotology- the study of the chemical properties of blood - it is not taught in medical schools. This is why your doctor won't know about treatments based on hemorheology.

And we believe that by changing aspects of how people who are depressed perceive and respond to the (often very depressing!) events in their lives—typically, feeling inappropriately guilty and responsible—you can change the person's internal chemistry, thus improving blood flow.

Les's contribution is a review of a range of scientific and medical definitions and hypotheses about depression, treatment approaches, and the role of cerebral blood flow in depression. This includes reports of cerebral blood flow problems observed in depressed patients, and the fact that these reports have largely been downplayed or ignored. There are life-style changes and easily obtainable supplements and drugs that can improve blood flow, and could therefore be expected to improve mood in depressed patients. The fact that this information is overlooked by the medical profession means that people who are depressed are not offered some treatments that could help them.

Les's work is written in the form and style of a scientific review. It will be challenging for most of us who are unfamiliar with this kind of writing, but very useful for readers who want to delve more deeply into the subject.

The book therefore begins with the first section of Les's work, followed with a section by Nancy on ways we can take charge of our depressing thoughts. The book continues in this form, interspersing our contributions.

Because most of this information won't be familiar to your doctor, counsellor, or therapist, you may have to become an ambassador for these ideas if they seem to make sense to you. When it comes to medical suggestions, these can only be undertaken under the supervision of your doctor.

WHAT LES TELLS US:
THE ROLE OF CEREBRAL BLOOD FLOW

A feature of the extensive literature dealing with depressive illness is the lack of reference to any of the many studies which report reduced rates of cerebral blood flow during episodes of depression. But even in those studies which report reduced regional cerebral blood flow in patients with major depressive disorder (MDD) there is no discussion concerning what factor or factors might be responsible for the observed reductions in blood flow. Possibly this is because the relevant medical science (hemorheology) is not taught at medical schools and appears to get little support from the major medical journals. In addition, because of the associated citation bias[2], it is not recognised that the reduced rate of regional cerebral blood flow might be treated by agents which improve blood rheology. But until the blood flow problems are recognised and dealt with, the management of depressive illness will be less than best.

---

[2] **Nancy:** *'Citation bias' refers to the fact that research papers are evaluated on how many times they are cited in other articles. The effect of this is that important information, if ignored, can disappear from the scientific radar, while trivial or even false information can gain credibility if a small group of researchers collaborate in citing each other's work.*

Depressive illness is a major health problem, worldwide, and plays an important role in suicides. MDD is subdivided into different types such as dysthymia, post-partum depression, seasonal disorder, but is different from bipolar depression. In the 21st century, those searching for information about the cause of depression would turn to the internet. For that reason, the following statements from different websites are of interest.

1. **Center for addiction and mental health.** "There is no simple answer to what causes depression, because several factors may play a part in the onset of the disorder. These include: a genetic or family history of depression, psychological or emotional vulnerability to depression, biological factors, and life events or environmental stressors."

2. **emedicinehealth.** "The causes of depression are complex. Genetic, biological and environmental factors can contribute to its development. In some people, depression can be traced to a single cause, while in others, a number of causes are at play. For many, the causes are never known."

3. **Everybody-health information for New Zealanders.** "The exact cause of depression is unknown. There is evidence to suggest that depression is an illness. There are also many theories regarding further aspects of this diverse condition. Different causes may operate in different people. This may be why there is variation in the way depression develops, in the symptoms and in the course."

4. **Family Doctor.org** "Depression seems to be related to a chemical imbalance in the brain which makes it hard for the cells to communicate with one another. Depression also seems to be hereditary (to run in families). Depression can be linked to stressful events in your life, such as the death of someone you love, a divorce or loss of your job. Taking

certain medicines, abusing drugs or alcohol or having other illnesses can also lead to depression."

5. **Health/Patient UK.** "The exact cause is not known. Anyone can become depressed. Some people are more prone to it, and it can develop for no apparent reason. You may have no particular problem or worry, but symptoms can develop quite suddenly. An episode of depression can also be triggered by a life event such as a relationship problem, bereavement, redundancy, illness, etc. For example, the combination of a mild low mood with some life problem, such as work stress, may lead to a spiral down to depression."

6. **Mayoclinic.com** "It's not known exactly what causes depression. As with many mental illnesses, it appears a variety of factors may be involved. These include;

- Biological differences. People with depression appear to have physical changes in their brains. The significance of these changes is still uncertain but may eventually help to pinpoint causes.

- Neurotransmitters. These naturally occurring brain chemicals linked to mood are thought to play a direct role in depression.

- Hormones. Changes in the body's balance of hormones may be involved in causing or triggering depression. Hormone changes can result from thyroid problems, menopause and a number of other conditions.

- Inherited traits. Depression is more common in people whose biological family members also have the condition. Researchers are still trying to find genes that may be involved in causing depression.

- Life events. Events such as the death or loss of a loved one, financial problems, and high stress can trigger depression in some people.

- Early childhood trauma. Traumatic events in childhood, such as abuse or loss of a parent may cause permanent changes in the brain that make you more susceptible to depression."

7. **Medline Plus Medical Encyclopedia.** "Depression often runs in families. This may be due to your genes (inherited), learned behaviour or both. Even if your genes make you more likely to develop depression, a stressful or unhappy life event usually triggers the onset of a depressive episode."

8. **National Institute of Mental Health.** "There is no single known cause of depression. Rather, it likely results from a combination of genetic, biochemical, environmental and psychological factors. Research indicates that depressive illnesses are disorders of the brain. Brain imaging technologies such as magnetic resonance imaging (MRI) have shown that the brains of people who have depression look different than those of people without depression. The parts of the brain responsible for regulating mood, thinking, sleep, appetite and behaviour appear to function abnormally. In addition, important neurotransmitters—chemicals that brain cells use to communicate—appear to be out of balance. But these images do not reveal why depression occurred. Some types of depression appear to run in families, suggesting a genetic link....... In addition, trauma, loss of a loved one, a difficult relationship or any stressful situation may trigger a depressive episode. Subsequent depressive episodes may occur with or without an obvious trigger."

9. **www.medicalnewstoday.** "We are still not sure what causes depression. Experts say depression is caused by a combination of factors, such as a person's genes, his biochemical environment, his personal experience and psychological factors. MRI (magnetic resonance imaging)

has shown that the brain of a person with depression looks different, compared to the brain of a person who has never had depression. The areas of the brain that deal with thinking, sleep, mood, appetite and behaviour do not appear to function normally. There are also indications that neurotransmitters appear to be out of balance.......We know that if there is depression in a family a person's chance of developing depression are higher......An awful experience can trigger a depressive illness. For example, the loss of a family member, a difficult relationship, physical or sexual abuse."

Thus nine authoritative websites are in general agreement, that not only is the cause of depression unknown, but also the mechanisms by which various triggering events stimulate an episode of depression are unexplained. Therefore it is surprising that none of these websites made reference to any of the 379 studies published between 1986 and 2010 in which single photon emission tomography (SPECT) was used to demonstrate reduced regional cerebral blood flow in patients with depressive disorder. The lack of recognition of those studies implies that citation bias has been operating for some time, although it would be surprising if normal brain function would persist in regions with reduced blood flow.

A SESSION WITH NANCY:
PERSONAL BOUNDARIES - HOW THEY WORK IN DEPRESSION

WHAT DO YOU TAKE IN?
WHAT DO YOU SEND OUT?

Imagine that we are sitting in the comfortable living-room which doubles as the place where I see clients.

We are sitting, facing each other, about seven or eight feet apart, you on the settee and I on a matching chair. The distance feels quite comfortable. If I move closer, we both begin to feel a bit tense, as though I am beginning to invade your personal space. If I move further away, it also feels uncomfortable, as though we are 'too far apart' for a relaxed conversation.

In fact, if we reach out our hands, we both can almost sense a point at which the boundaries of 'my personal space' and 'your personal space' meet.

There are many ways in which this concept can be used in a therapeutic situation, but let's just stay with how it tends to work in depression.

Imagine that this boundary, this edge, marks the space within which everything is 'you' and outside of which everything is 'not you'. Now imagine that this has a tough, transparent protective layer, so that you can see anything coming toward you, and make a decision about whether to let it in or keep it out.

Now I ask you 'If someone says something critical about you, do you believe it is true?' Most usually, if you are depressed, you agree—so you let this negative comment come in. You believe it is true, and it helps to confirm your bad feelings about yourself.

What about compliments, praise? 'Oh no, I never believe it when someone says something nice about me.' So, positive comments are stopped at the border—shut out. The good feelings which the person giving you a compliment wants to transmit are blocked out—left on the doorstep!

OK, now, do you ever say anything critical to other people? 'No, of course not.'

Do you get cross when people are nasty to you? 'I might feel bad, but I'd never say anything nasty back.' Your negative feelings are kept within the border, not fired out towards others.

And do you ever praise or compliment other people? 'Oh yes, I always try to be nice to other people.' Your positive feelings, your good will, are projected outwards towards others. However bad you may be feeling, you try to make other people feel good.

Can you see how this leaves all the negative feelings inside your personal boundary, and keeps anything that would make you feel better outside? No wonder it feels bad in there!

So let's have a rethink about this whole situation.

First of all, let's be realistic about criticism. Sometimes a person who has your best interests at heart will want to help you improve what you are doing, in your job, your relationships, or your other activities, and they will point out something that you are doing wrong. Criticism can contain information that can be useful to you. If intended with good will, and also accurate, such criticism can be a useful guide to action.

However, if people are feeling upset or put upon or frustrated about their own situations, they may lash out, as a way of making someone else feel bad so they can feel better. Their criticism (or nastiness) *is information about how they are feeling,* **not** information about you. That sort of criticism can safely be left outside your personal boundary.

Most criticism that makes us feel bad is, when you think about it, that sort of thing. If it is about another person's frustration, then they have a problem that they need to solve. If their response is just to try to pass their frustration on to someone else, by lashing out at them, they won't solve their problem. Letting them make you feel bad instead of using their frustration as a cue to sort out their own problem is like accepting a package that doesn't belong to you. And like a parcel that has been sent to the wrong address, you do not need to accept it. So when criticism comes you way, stop it at the boundary, have a look at it. Then decide whether it is accurate about you (maybe you have been in late three times this week and need to do something about it) or information about the sender (she came in looking like a thunder-cloud, and everyone knew she was going to have a go at someone). Just because she is feeling bad doesn't mean you have to. Offering her sympathy might be a more appropriate response than allowing the fact that she's feeling bad to make you feel bad. If someone has the habit of making others suffer instead of dealing with the issues in their own life, the kindest thing is to decline to suffer, leaving the problem where it belongs. She may decide to deal with it, she may not, but at least when you refuse to take on her bad feelings, you are giving her the chance to do something more constructive.

Now let's look at compliments, praise. What reason would someone have for telling you that they like your blouse/hair cut/smile, or say that you've done a good job, or that they admire some personal quality of yours, other than that they do? If they are trying to win a favour, or sell you something, or get you into bed, maybe that is the reason. If none of those apply, why would a person bother to say something nice unless it was because that is what they genuinely believe? And they like you well enough to want to tell you so? When that comes towards you, let it in! (And maybe you should let it in anyway—you can still enjoy the compliment without having to do the favour, buy anything, or go to bed with someone you don't fancy!)

Warding off compliments ('oh, this old thing?' 'I think I look dreadful' 'it wasn't anything') will be a habit so ingrained that you probably don't even notice you are doing it. But how do you feel when you say something nice to someone and they brush it off? It's a bit of an emotional slap in the face. So why do that to others….change your ways! Take compliments as most likely to be information about you—accurate information. This parcel has been sent to the right address. So smile, say 'thank you', and accept it. (As your teenager would say, Get Used to It!)

What about sending out negative stuff—criticisms, nastiness? I know that you don't want to do that, and I would not suggest that you do. But if you thought that someone was doing something really dangerous, I am sure you wouldn't hesitate to shout 'stop', or 'look out'. Maybe when you consider the people around you from a realistic perspective, you will recognise that there is information that could sound critical, but which they would benefit from, and you will want to consider the best way for them to get that information. That isn't sent from a place of wanting to be hurtful.

But when something hurtful comes in your direction, and it is about some unresolved problem in someone else's life, you don't want to retaliate, but it is their package, not yours—leave it outside—allow yourself to consider it calmly and with compassion. They will never solve their own problems if they simply resort to taking it out on others. You are not doing them any favours by allowing them to make you feel bad.

We need to think about our personal boundaries another way. If we are depressed, it often goes with not feeling as though we have the right to say 'No' to anyone, even if unreasonable demands are being made on our attention, time, effort or money. If our resources are being drained, we are going to feel 'low'. Negotiating our right to limit the claims of others may be an issue that we need help with. A good guess is that women find this harder to do, because nature has designed us to deal with the one situation in which unlimited claims are justified—the needs of a newborn. If the person making unreasonable demands is not an infant, then you may need practical, as well as psychological help in dealing with your situation. This applies whether this is an older child, a spouse, a parent, or a friend. The first step is to realise that you have a right to limit demands on you. The second will be finding ways to set those limits.

Often it is easier to tell people what you will do than what you won't do. To the friend who rings endlessly to complain about their situation but never accepts advice about how to change it, you could say 'You know, I'd love to hear about what you are going to do about it, so do ring me when you've decided what that will be.' If it's a person whom you feel has a right to your attention, set a definite time for a phone call or a visit. It doesn't have to be 'I don't want to speak to you/see you until Tuesday', it can be 'I'll be delighted to speak to you/see you on Tuesday'. An unwanted or inconvenient phone call can be met with 'You know, this is too important to be rushed, let's have a proper chat about it tomorrow at ......' (You specify the time and the length of the proper chat!) You will find other ways to sound warm and positive while taking control of the use of your time, energy, or resources. Often very demanding people are in the grip of some sort of addiction, even just an addiction to having problems....preferring problems to solutions! As above, encourage this person to talk to you about solutions. You wouldn't give an alcoholic money for a drink...but you could give encouragement to go to AA. If your demanding friend has a medical, legal, psychiatric or relationship problem, your involvement doesn't have to be more than advice to go to the appropriate professional. One of the perpetuating factors in depression is feeling you don't have the right not to meet everyone's demands, or the right to expect reciprocation. But you do—so stay with the friend who has time to listen to you, who pays you back money you lend, who will do you a favour back when you have done one for him/her, who takes your advice and thanks you for it. And if it is one way traffic, it is fine when that 'friend' finds someone else to put upon. As they will, once you start setting limits.

Of course, in today's political and economic climate, most of us are now supposed to accept a situation in which having a zero hours contract is called 'having a job', firms complain that paying a living wage is unaffordable, and we are encouraged to believe that disabled people are just lazy. Politically, it is acceptable for us to be placed in situations in which all of our efforts are not enough to provide us or our families with basic necessities. It's not surprising that a lot of us are depressed.

However, on the level of our everyday relationships, as you begin to leave the bad stuff outside, and let the good stuff come in, start setting limits on others' demands and recognise your right to reciprocation, you will be making a very important change in some of the mental habits that contribute to depression.

And maybe recognising that your depression has been encouraged by political and economic circumstances created by other people for their own benefit will lead you to exchange depression for some sort of political action!

LES CONTINUES:
THE PATHOPHYSIOLOGY OF DEPRESSIVE ILLNESS

As noted in the website extracts, the nature of the cause or causes of depressive illness remain unexplained. However, since the 1960s at least, there has been a vast number of theories published, and what follows is not an exhaustive account, but has the aim of demonstrating the diversity of opinion in this field. However, it should be noted that the first sentence of the abstract of a 2007 paper stated, *"The cause of mental disorders such as depression remains unknown."*

(a) Theories and hypotheses

An evolutionary theory considers depression to be a survival tactic that promotes the survival of the weaker members of society. A "malaise" theory suggests that, *"...the minimal or core state of depression, is a 'normal' brain's response to an abnormal body state."* It has been argued that MDD is inappropriate sickness behaviour, and that the syndrome of MDD is generated by abnormalities in cytokines. Therefore it was proposed that antidepressants exerted an analgesic effect. Such a concept is greatly different from that of the cognitive theory which postulated that the source of depression was the thought processes of the mind—which included sadness, loss of self esteem and hopelessness. In contrast, the psychoanalytic theory was based upon the importance of inter-personal relationships. A neurobiology theory deals with various neurotransmitters, particularly serotonin, norepinephrine and dopamine. The biopsychosocial model proposes that the three facets (biological, psychological, social) all contribute to the development of depression. However, there may be great variation in the contribution from each factor. Because depressive illness is frequent in the elderly, the vascular depression hypothesis proposes that vascular disease predisposes to and may perpetuate depression.

In the face of such a wide variety of concepts, it is very likely that the management and treatments offered for depression should be very variable. With the objective of obtaining a wider perspective, the published, relevant literature was surveyed.

This literature survey does not purport to be exhaustive, as more than 3000 titles were obtained from a PubMed search for "depressive illness." As a result, the selection of topics concerned those which had been the subject of many investigations, and to a large extent the various topics indicate the inherent problems which have inhibited an understanding of the etiopathogenesis of depressive illness. It is very likely that the diversity of viewpoints which mark the various theories, are, to a major extent, due to the lack of an accepted etiopathogenesis.

The situation is not clarified by the fact that depressive illness may co-exist with other medical problems which range from psychiatric illness to cardiovascular disorders, with claims that depression is a risk factor for those disorders. In the English translation of the abstract of a 2008 paper in German (1) the current situation was summarised as follows. *"Despite its clinical and socio-economic relevance, surprisingly little is known on the etiology of depression. A multitude of neurobiological and psychosocial hypotheses have been postulated but most lack empirical validity or cannot be integrated into comprehensive psychological models."*

(b) Cortisol levels

There has been much discussion about the implications of the hyperactivity of the hypothalamus-pituitary axis, with higher than usual levels of cortisol in depression. However, it has to be assumed that the measurement of cortisol levels in saliva, plasma and urine produce equivalent data. For example Vreeburg et al (2) compared saliva cortisol levels at one hour after wakening and in the evening in 308 controls; in 579 subjects with no current depressive disorder and 701 subjects with a diagnosis of MDD. Cortisol levels were higher than controls in both the current and remitted groups and were not affected by 0.5mg dexamethazone.

The higher levels of cortisol in the depressed and non-depressed groups were interpreted as being, *"...indicative of an increased biological vulnerability for depression."* However, according to Scharnholz et al (3), during acute episodes of depression, acutely depressed patients showed higher levels of cortisol excretion than controls, but in both fully and partially remitted patients, night time urine showed declining levels of cortisol excretion. That result is at odds with the findings of Vreeburg et al (2). As different studies assess cortisol levels differently, the findings are difficult to correlate. For example, Piwowarska et al (4) assessed the serum levels of cortisol before and during treatment with an antidepressant in a study of 17 patients with MDD. Plasma cortisol levels were assessed at time zero, 3 hours, 24 hours and at 4, 6 and 8 weeks. Eight MDD patients showed an average of 46% increase in cortisol levels. In 13 patients who responded to clonipramine, during 0-6 weeks, cortisol levels decreased. But in a study (5) in which salivary cortisol levels were assessed in 126 MDD patients 45 minutes after awakening and three times during the evening it was noted,

"Patient-reported shorter total sleep hours, more severe levels of depression and higher suffering levels were positively associated with flatter diurnal cortisol patterns." Furthermore, *"Severe levels of depression were more likely related to flatter diurnal cortisol patterns than moderate and mild levels of depression."* The results of such studies fail to clarify just what role cortisol might play in depressive disorder.

(c) Neurotransmitters

Other factors which are considered to be important in the hypothalamus-pituitary-adrenal axis, are the neurotransmitters serotonin, dopamine and norepinephrine. The postulated importance of serotonin has been recognised by the development of a series of drugs, the selective serotonin re-uptake inhibitors (SSRIs) which enhance neurotransmission by retaining serotonin in the synapse for longer than usual by inhibiting its re-uptake in the pre-synaptic cell. In addition, there are selective norepinephrine re-uptake inhibitors; selective serotonin-norepinephrine reuptake inhibitors and selective serotonin-norepinephrine-dopamine inhibitors. There are about seven of these drugs, two of which are sold under ten different trade names so SSRIs can be a source of confusion. But if neurotransmission suffered from synaptic problems then some of these drugs should be effective. Even though SSRIs and SNRIs are considered to be the first choice for treatment of MDD (6) their overall effects are unimpressive. A large number of side effects may occur during the first four weeks of therapy. Even though the SSRIs have been in use for more than 20 years, their ineffectiveness has been reported frequently with discontinuation of the drug in 1-4 weeks because of ineffectiveness or due to side effects. For that reason, there are many reports of the effects of other antidepressant drugs in the 30-50% of patients who failed to respond to SSRIs. Faravelli et al (7) found in a small study that tricyclic antidepressants were more effective than SSRIs, but in contrast, meta-analyses published by Geddes et al in 2000 (8) and in 2007 (9) concluded that, *"There are no clinically significant differences in effectiveness between selective serotonin re-uptake inhibitors and tricyclic antidepressants. Treatment decisions need to be based on considerations of relative patient acceptability, toxicity and cost."* Although SSRIs are used as primary treatment for MDD their ineffectiveness has led to many trials of SSRIs and with other medications. For example, Trivedi et al (10) studied the effects of sustained release bupropion and buspirone in MDD patients who had failed to reach remission after treatment with citalopram—an SSRI. Between 25% and 40% of patients responded to the medications. More recently, a study in Mexico (11) compared the effects of an SSRI and an SNRI. Both groups showed an improved memory and other functions, but cognitive function failed to reach that of controls.

What seems most apparent, is that despite a very large number of published studies, the basis for treatment of MDD which is aimed at prolonging the time that neurotransmitters spend in the synapse, seems to be of dubious value.

(d) Cytokines

In 2001, Leonard (12) published an interesting paper titled, "Changes in the immune system in depression and dementia: cause or co-incidental effects ?" He claimed that, *"In major depression, evidence is provided to show both activation (eg macrophage activity, acute phase proteins) and inhibition (eg natural killer cell activity) of the immune system occurs."* But two years later, Steptoe et al (13) assessed the indicators of immune activation and vascular inflammation in 122 men and 104 women aged 47-59 years. They reported, *"There were no associations between the measures of depressive symptoms and hopelessness and markers of immune activation or of inflammatory response."* The authors concluded, *"...disturbances of immune function and inflammatory processes are unlikely to be primarily responsible for the association between depressive symptoms and coronary heart disease."* Schiepers et al (14) noted, *"The cytokine hypothesis of depression implies that the pro-inflammatory cytokines acting on neuromodulators, represent the key factor in the central mediation of the behavioural, neuroendocrine, and neurochemical features of depressive disorder."* After discussing various aspects of the hypothesis, the authors concluded, *"...it remains to be established whether cytokines play a causal role in depressive illness or represent epiphenomena without major significance."* This uncertainty about the relevance of cytokines in the development of depressive illness was reflected in a report of the relevance of animal studies (15) which concluded, *"However, cytokines do not appear to be essential mediators of depressive illness."* To a considerable extent, the findings of Marques-Doak et al (16) mirror the findings of Steptoe et al (13) when they reported that, *"Patients currently depressed, had similar levels of cytokines and cortisol as healthy controls."* The English abstract of a Portugese meta-analysis (17) concluded, *"Cytokines MAY (my emphasis) play a role in the pathophysiology of SOME (my emphasis) cases of depression, although a causal link has not been established yet."*

Thus, on the basis of the published information, it would seem that the measurable aspects of the cytokine hypothesis of MDD are not supported by actual measurements and for that reason are unlikely to be a cause of MDD.

(e) Vascular depression hypothesis

This topic has been chosen for discussion as it seems to exemplify the problems which can arise from citation bias. In 1997, Alexopoulos et al (18) proposed that, *"...cerebrovascular disease may predispose, precipitate or perpetuate some geriatric depressive syndromes."* The authors claimed that the hypothesis, *"...is supported by the comorbidity of depression, vascular disease and vascular risk factors and the association of ischaemic lesions to distinctive behavioural symptoms.*" However, the failure to recognise the implications of many reports concerning reduced regional cerebral blood flow as a causal factor in depression is surprising, and the term "reduced cerebral blood flow" occurs only once in the text, on p916. This was in the statement, "*In asymptomatic patients, white matter hyperintensities were found to be associated with extracranial carotid artery disease, reduced cerebral blood flow, and a history of hypertension, diabetes and cardiac disease.*" As the increased tissue water content demonstrated by white matter hyperintensities could be a manifestation of the effects of increased blood viscosity on the extravasation of water from capillaries, it should be noted that there are many reports which show that hypertension, diabetes and cardiac disease share the common feature of increased blood viscosity which will reduce the rate of blood flow. Furthermore, there is published evidence that myocardial infarction can occur in the absence of vascular disease. Fournier et al (19) reported that 27 of 87 patients who had survived despite being heavy smokers, had, "*...angiographically normal coronary arteries.*" It is possible that the smoking-related increase in blood viscosity could have been the causal factor. As a similar finding of normal coronary arteries in patients who had heart attacks, was reported in a 2001 study, it is not essential for vascular disease to be a factor in myocardial infarction.

In their definition of vascular depression, the cardinal features were as follows. "Clinical and/or laboratory evidence of vascular disease or vascular risk factors. Clinical manifestations may include history of stroke or transient ischaemic attacks, focal neurological signs, atrial fibrillation, angina, history of myocardial infarction, carotid bruit, hypertension and hyperlipidaemia. Laboratory findings may include significant white matter hyperintensities at the territory of the perforating arteries, infarcts, or evidence of carotid occlusion or stenosis of the Willis circle arteries." It is noteworthy that there is no mention of blood viscosity-reduced blood flow, as there are many published reports of increased blood viscosity playing a causal role in myocardial infarction, hypertension and in hyperlipidemic situations. The effects of age were introduced as follows. *"Depression onset after 65 years of age or change in the cause of depression after the onset of vascular disease in patients with early-onset depression: development of more frequent and persistent depressive episodes."* But the age-related increases in blood viscosity were not mentioned and the blood flow problems were interpreted as consequences of vascular disease.

> ***Nancy:*** *Here, as in many other places, Les is pointing out that blood flow problems are almost invariably considered to be 'vascular', that is, having to do with the blood vessels, rather than to do with blood viscosity—the limits imposed on flow due to the increase in shape-changed, non-deformable red blood cells.*

Thus the cardinal features of the hypothesis draw attention to the fundamental problems which have followed on from a selective use of the published information. For example, in the search of the published literature, how would it have been possible to miss a title such as, "Cerebral blood flow in depression," (20) which was published in a major journal? Furthermore, in 1980 (21) and in 1995 (22) there were other reports concerning cerebral blood flow and depression. For example, the conclusion of Mathew et al (21) was that, *"Marked reductions in regional cerebral blood flow correlated significantly with depth of depression as measured by the Hamilton Depression Scale."* Perhaps the strangest example of citation bias concerns their references 71 and 72, both of which are studies of regional cerebral blood flow from the English group headed by CJ Bench, and published in 1992. However, no reference was made to the 1995 paper from the group (23) which concluded, *"Thus recovery from depression is associated with increases in regional cerebral blood flow in the same area in which decreases in regional cerebral blood flow are described in the depressed state, in comparison with normal subjects."* **This observation implies that remissions are associated with the normalisation of the flow properties of the blood as it is very unlikely that vascular diseases could have been cured so quickly. In addition, the association of improved blood flow with an absence of depression could explain the mechanism of the benefits of inter-personal therapies such as psychotherapy. The calming influence of counselling would lower the level of the stress hormones, thus restoring the red cell environment to normal, increasing red cell deformability and improving blood flow.**

Nancy: This is the point at which Les' information that improved blood flow can help alleviate depression and how psychotherapy can improve blood flow intersects with the knowledge that some forms of psychotherapy can alleviate depression.

The cardinal feature concerning the onset of depression after 65 years of age is another indication of citation bias as it implies a rejection of published studies concerning the aging process. As the blood flow patterns of those 65 years of age and older are quite different from those 50 years of age and younger, it is not possible to generalise from observations made on the over-65 group. In 1974 (24) it was reported that blood viscosity was lower in subjects aged between 12 and 29 years than that of subjects aged between 69 and 91 years. The authors noted that, *"The tendency for blood viscosity to be greater at low shear rates probably reflected the presence of poorly deformable red cells."* That observation was in agreement with the results of an unpublished study of blood samples from 315 healthy subjects aged between 40 and 79 years. The blood samples were assessed by viscometry and filtration through 5micron pores to obtain a measure of red cell deformability. Blood from those aged 60 years and older was more viscous and less filterable than that of those aged 59 years and younger. But a small number of subjects in their 40s had results similar to those over 60 years of age. Those findings had implications for other published studies concerning cerebral blood flow. A Swedish study of cerebral blood flow in 87 subjects aged between 19 and 68 years, (25) concluded, *"...the mean cerebral blood flow decreased progressively with age."* Similarly, a British study of regional cerebral blood flow in 30 normal volunteers aged between 30 and 80 years, concluded, *"Decreases in regional cerebral blood flow suggest a regionally specific loss of cerebral function with age."* (26)

Thus, prior to the publication of the vascular depression hypothesis, there was published evidence that the aged had increased blood viscosity and reduced red cell deformability. As such changes reduce the rate of blood flow it is not surprising that increasing age was associated with reductions in regional cerebral blood flow.

In an invited commentary titled, "The vascular depression hypothesis: 10 years later," (27) Alexopoulos claimed that, *"Almost 10 years later, one can argue that the vascular depression hypothesis has served the field well in providing research direction."* In order to obtain some measure of research interest in the field of the hypothesis, I carried out a PubMed search for, "the vascular depression hypothesis in humans" which produced 186 titles. However 33 of those titles were published prior to the publication of the hypothesis in 1997. Most of the papers dealt with other hypotheses (106 papers) while 31 papers supported the hypothesis and the results of 12 studies did not support it. But some of the 31 supporting papers came from members of the group which published the 1997 paper, and another group published 5 studies which claimed their results supported the hypothesis. Therefore given the relative paucity of studies, it is arguable as to whether or not the hypothesis, *"...has served the field well in providing research direction."* It should be noted that none of the 153 abstracts assessed made any reference to the literature concerning cerebral blood flow and depression.

> **Nancy:** *The results of the literature search described above demonstrate the power of citation bias: the claim that the vascular depression hypothesis 'has served the field well', once one has made a careful study of the supposedly supportive papers, is shown to be based on very flimsy grounds indeed.*

The general failure to recognise a possible role for changed blood rheology in the pathogenesis of depressive illness is epitomised by an example given by Alexopoulos. He referred to a young woman who developed depression after a family separation, suffered from post-partum depression, and who also suffered *"...a new depressive episode following a frontolimbic insult late in life."* All 3 episodes of depression could be the expected outcome of changes in the internal environment which would give rise to shape-changed, poorly-deformable red cells which would contribute to increased blood viscosity and reduced rates of blood flow.[3]

In contrast to the 1997 paper there is no mention of blood flow, but it is relevant that in 1998 a paper from the US National Institute on Aging (28) cited 82 references in reporting that increasing blood viscosity and reducing red cell deformability are parts of the normal aging process. So in electing to work with people aged 65 years and older, the authors of the hypothesis had chosen a group whose members would show variable changes in blood rheology. This ensured that it was not possible to extrapolate from their findings to younger groups with normal blood rheology.

Therefore, it seems reasonable to conclude that the citation bias which was a feature of the 1997 paper, was still in vogue ten years later.

It is concluded that none of this material can satisfactorily explain the nature of relapsing/remitting depressive illness, which is consistent with he views expressed in websites which claim that the cause of depression is unknown. This implies that in the absence of an accepted etiopathogenesis, the treatment of depression will be less than best.

---

[3] **Nancy:** *A excellent example of the range of events which could lead to depression: in the first, an emotional response to a separation, in the second, a response to hormonal imbalances after giving birth, the third a physiological response to a head injury. Each would affect the chemical environment within the blood, resulting in shape changes in the red blood cells. Here, in the first example, psychotherapy would be helpful, in the second, addressing the hormonal imbalance, in the third, appropriate medical care. In all examples, measures to improve blood flow could be expected to be effective in treating the depression.*

BACK TO NANCY:
BANDLER'S IMPERTINENT QUESTION

NOT 'WHY', BUT 'HOW'

Surely the question to ask me, as a person who is depressed, is 'why'? Traditional therapy asks the patient to talk about all the events in their lives that have added up to 'making them' depressed. Traditional therapy makes the assumption that if you go back to your bad memories, re-experience them as fully and realistically as possible, this will somehow enable you to work through, to overcome their emotional effects. Unfortunately, it often has the opposite effect, simply reinforcing the emotions you experienced at the time, as well as some negative beliefs about yourself that probably go along with them.

The neglected or abused child is likely to feel that being ignored or mistreated is a punishment—they must have done something to deserve it. Tragically, rather than coming to believe that the adults who should be caring for them are doing wrong, most often children learn to feel that whatever is going on must be their fault—and the worse it is, the worse they feel about themselves. These beliefs, this 'victim guilt', are a prominent feature in depression—as many of the descriptions Les has shown us point out, *inappropriate guilt and self-criticism are characteristic symptoms.* It can be one of the most difficult issues for a therapist to help a person resolve. I will come to my ideas about why this is, and what we can do about it, later on.

A person who is depressed may be able to provide a very detailed and poignant answer to the traditional therapeutic question—'why'. Losing a parent at an early age, being rejected or humiliated as a child, having a mother too depressed or ill herself to engage with her child, witnessing violence in the family and feeling helpless to prevent it are among the recurring themes in the lives of people who suffer from depression.[4] But too often, recounting these events to a psychotherapist doesn't lead to a change in the person's state of mind—often, it can simply reinforce it. This is because 'reliving' an experience—remembering as if we were 'back in it'—brings back the emotions and the accompanying beliefs. This can be avoided, and we'll explain further on about how a therapist using neurolinguistic methods can help their client do this.

In the meantime, back to Bandler and his impertinent question to the person who is depressed - which is: 'How are you doing that?'

It seems impertinent because if you ask a person how they are doing something, it seems to imply that they are doing something knowingly and on purpose. No one would knowingly and on purpose inflict the suffering of depression on themselves, and that isn't what he is implying. He points out that, unlike your new car, our brain doesn't come with an instruction manual. He tries to provide us with one. Figuring out how our brain 'does' depression gives us a handle on how

---

[4] Louis Cozolino, in his book 'The Neuroscience of Human Relationships - Attachment and the Developing Social Brain' (W.W. Norton & Co, New York, 2006, ISBN 13: 978-0-393-70454-9) gives a detailed, extremely well-documented account of the way early experiences affect the physiological development of the brain, with significant implications for subsequent mental health.

we might change that, much as our car's instruction manual might tell us what to do when the car stalls.

So what is the answer? What, exactly, is our brain doing, that is making us feel so bad?

This is an example from an early chapter of his book 'Using Your Brain for a Change'.[5] He watched a young woman at a party, having a wonderful time, for three hours. Just as she was about to leave, she spilled a cup of coffee on her dress. She burst into tears, exclaiming 'That's ruined my whole evening!' Bandler asked her to explain to him what was going on in her mind as she made this statement. The young woman realised that she was visualising her memories of the party, seeing them as though the coffee stain had been on her dress the whole time.

Bandler believes that we can understand all sorts of emotional distress (as well as the processes of feeling happy, and the processes of performing at the highest level in activities such as sports, or music) if we examine the elements of how we 'think', or 'mentally represent' activities and events.

Our language is full of metaphors that indicate an implicit understanding of this view. We speak of memories 'fading', of being able to 'look back and laugh', or being able to recall a memory 'as though it is happening all over again'.

The word 'depression' can denote a range of feelings from being 'slightly blue' or 'under the weather', to being

---

[5] 'Using Your Brain For A Change', Richard Bandler, Real People Press, U.S., 1 August 1985, ISBN-10-0091122623, ISBN-13-98-091122620. All of the information about NLP in this book originated in the writings of Richard Bandler and John Grinder, and since has been widely disseminated by other authors. Some of the specific techniques mentioned have been developed through my own practice.

completely incapacitated by a profound combination of sadness and guilt. The symptom mentioned most frequently, along with sadness, melancholy, gloom, is self-criticism— which again can range from obsessing about relatively minor failings and misdeeds, to delusions of having caused deaths and disasters on a grand scale.

(In case the reader is tempted to dismiss the latter as just being silly, or absolutely crazy, consider all the historical accounts, for example the Biblical account of Noah and the flood, in which natural disasters have been coded as the result of the sins of the people, literally 'the wrath of God'.)

In order to begin to understand how we can take charge of ways that we think, we first need to look in more detail about how our brain processes information.

REPRESENTATIONAL SYSTEMS

We experience the world through our five senses—seeing, hearing, 'feeling' (either a physical sensation or emotion), smelling, tasting. We 'think' using the same five senses—in mental pictures, sounds (including words and music), feelings (the sensation of diving into a chilly pool, or enjoying the first warmth of spring), and smells and tastes, either remembered or imagined.

We may remember our last holiday, and some of us will think first of the sights we saw, while others will remember how hot or how cold the weather was, and others the sounds we heard—waves breaking, an unfamiliar language, the local music. Or the unfamiliar smells, the taste of the local food. When we are planning to go to somewhere new, we will imagine what it will be like, creating or constructing the images, the sounds and sensations we may be going to encounter.

So there are fifteen, more or less, ways we can be directing our attention: we can be actually looking at, or listening to, or feeling, smelling or tasting something in our environment (Perceiving, external). We can be remembering something seen, heard, felt, smelt or tasted. (Remembering, internal.) Or we can be imagining something that we will be seeing, hearing, feeling, smelling, or tasting, in the future. (Constructing—imagining—, internal.)

All of our activities can be described as sequences of these categories. For example, when we are driving a car, we need to be looking outside the car or in the mirrors—visual, external. We also need to be listening, both to sounds from outside the car, and the sounds that the car is making. (Auditory, external) And we need to be using our physical memory of the correct hand movements for changing gears and using the handbrake, or foot movements to reach the controls in order to clutch, brake or accelerate without having to look down. (Kinesthetic, remembered—internal, then performed—external.)

There is a more detailed, diagrammatic explanation of representational systems in the Appendix.

There is a special mental process which is different from the others, which we call 'internal dialogue' (or 'talking to ourselves'!). Most often, this is self-critical—I have never encountered anyone whose internal dialogue is constantly reiterating how attractive, good, talented they are (if there are such people, they probably don't need to come for therapy!). My guess is that this is because it has a protective function, and perhaps the critical content is some memory of things our parents said (or shouted) to us when they were either frightened for us or angry at us. After all, survival is more likely if the child about to go out in a busy road responds to 'Stop! Don't do that! Be careful! Don't be silly!' and there are many other situations in which our parents will know it is important for our safety, our social acceptance, our education, to obey the rules.

However, there are degrees and degrees of criticism and punishment. The modern, educated parent is supposed to know that there is an important distinction to be made between criticising the child's behaviour, and criticising the child herself. Hopefully, as a child, I will learn that I am valued and loved, even though some of my behaviour is naughty. If my parents are depressed and unresponsive, or constantly angry, or actively abusive, I become more likely to come to believe that I am intrinsically a bad person. The more severe the abuse, the more I become convinced that I must be terribly evil, or this wouldn't be happening. (And abuse often includes being told that I am thoroughly bad or evil.)

However it would be a mistake to focus solely on what parents do. Family misfortunes, deaths, accidents, illness, even financial stresses can create atmospheres in which a young child may begin to experience not only grief, but anxiety about what might happen, and wondering if any of it might be the child's fault, in the same way we all question whether, if we had done things better, misfortunes may not have occurred.

The internal dialogue of a depressed person is typically extremely self-critical, full of reasons to think unkindly of themselves, to believe they are incompetent, stupid, unattractive, undeserving, fundamentally unlovable. In psychotic depression, these thoughts become really extreme. The degree and intensity of such feelings are likely to be an accurate measure of how extreme the events are which has led to them. (A client once said to me that in his childhood, he was glad to wake up from having been knocked unconscious by his father—that meant a good day, because his Dad wouldn't be doing it again at least for a little while.)

Children who witness domestic violence, or experience the loss of a parent, or are in a family experiencing mental health problems or material hardship also are likely to grow up with a mistaken idea that there must have been something they could have done to make things better, and to have a deep sense of failure.

So, to recap, we use our five senses to perceive things externally. When we are 'thinking', what we are doing is using our five senses inside our head—remembering, or imagining, pictures; sounds (including music or words); feelings (either physical sensations or emotions); smells; and tastes. And we also experience a stream of inner comment (internal dialogue) which is usually more critical than reassuring. Paradoxically, the worse a time we have had in our lives, the more critical this tends to be. Sadly, rather than being critical of the people or the events that harmed us when we were children, it turns the criticism onto ourself.

As an adult, looking back at those experiences, we can see more clearly where power and responsibility lay, and begin to feel appropriately sympathetic toward the child that we were. As we do that, our internal critical voice can begin to soften, and to tell us more accurate things. After all, we were children in a tough situation, we found ways to survive. We were brave, caring, and desperate to improve matters over which we had no control. How admirable is that?

More about these two processes later. Back to the simple things!

EYE MOVEMENTS THAT GIVE US AWAY![6]

When we are just 'thinking', it is possible for someone watching us to tell whether we are thinking in pictures, words, feelings, or internal dialogue. When we are remembering a scene, our eyes will be gazing up and to the left. If we are

---

[6] Bandler, Richard (1979). *Frogs into princes: neuro linguistic programming*. Moab, Utah: Real People Press. ISBN 978-0-911226-19-5.

trying to picture something we haven't yet seen (where we will be on our next holiday), our gaze will be up to the right.

If we are 'thinking' in sound (auditory), our gaze will mostly be level, to the left if we are remembering, to the right if we are thinking about what we are going to say next. (Remember the 'shifty-eyed foreigner'? He, or she, is trying to remember how to say things in the new language, and then imagining saying them—eyes level, swinging from right to left and back again.)

If we are thinking about or remembering something physical that we did (diving into a pool, for example), our gaze will be down to our right. This will also be the case if what we are feeling is an emotion. When we are deep in internal dialogue, our eyes will be down, to the left.

To see this clearly, have a look at the diagram of eye movements in the Appendix.

There are also typical postures and breathing patterns which go along with these mental states. A person who is highly visual will also have an erect posture, and shallow breathing, high in the chest. The person preoccupied with sound will be less erect, breathing from the mid chest. The person mainly dwelling in feelings is likely to be looking down, sitting with a curved spine, breathing from the abdomen.

Now that people with even quite serious mental health problems are mostly living in the community, you may remember seeing someone you can just tell is very depressed: carelessly dressed, walking slowly along, with a bowed head, looking at the pavement, evidently muttering to him or herself.

The simple answer to 'how' people who are depressed are 'doing it', is that they are 'listening to' intensely self-critical internal dialogue, believing that it is true, and feeling very bad.

If you have come for help about your depression, you will be talking to me in slow, measured tones, looking at the floor, and will be saying things about yourself that you wouldn't think of saying to anyone else—'I'm just stupid, I'm wasting your time, I've done such terrible things, it was my fault that it all happened'. I know that there would be no point in my disagreeing with you, or trying to talk you out of it.

So, instead, I will ask you to sit up straight, take a couple of breaths, and fix your gaze on a point slightly below the ceiling. Now I will ask you whether you can keep your gaze fixed upward like that, and feel depressed at the same time, without letting your gaze drop. ('And notice what happens when you blink!') You will be surprised to discover that it isn't possible.

Keeping an upward direction of gaze, and the corresponding posture, simply blocks the neural connections involved in depression. We are an integrated system—our physiological position and state, our thoughts, and the chemistry in our body are all interlinked—which means that if you can find a way to break a link, you can break up the whole process. It isn't easy to change strong and persistent habits of thought, belief, posture and mood. But it is easy to move your eyeballs about a centimetre! It will take longer to persuade you that you are an intrinsically good person, and that you weren't responsible for your parents' divorce, your grandmother's death, or the state of the world, but this is a start.

The first stage, in tackling depression through simple physical means, then, is to persuade you to start looking up a lot. I think that if there is some way to position TV screens, and PC monitors so that your gaze is upward, that would help. When you are outdoors, concentrate (after making sure you aren't going to trip over anything, or go in front of a car) on studying the rooflines of the houses, the tops of trees, the cloud formations in the sky. The phrase 'uplifting' has real significance here! As you make this into a permanent habit, you will find that your mood becomes correspondingly lighter.

To recap: If we think about the fifteen 'areas of attention', we find that the processes of depression include the physical act of looking down, and the internal processes of paying attention to self-critical internal dialogue, and feeling bad, sad and guilty! One way of short-circuiting this is to change the direction of our gaze, look up at what is out there; shift our attention from internal to external, and to whatever is visible when we direct our gaze upward—rooflines of houses, the tops of trees, clouds in the sky. For as long as we can resist the downward pull of depressive thought processes, and keep our gaze physically upward, we will not be able to experience the feelings of depression at the same time. It is worth taking time and effort to practice shifting our attention in this way, until it begins to replace the habit of looking down and feeling 'low'!

(Don't be too surprised to find you just don't want to! That's the depression talking!)

And of course, life is not this simple—we need more strategies for cutting through these negative loops of thought-feeling-thought. More precisely, internal self-criticism—guilt—self-criticism. Take some time to practice 'looking up'. We'll deal with internal dialogue and victim guilt later. In the meantime, back to Les.

BACK TO LES:
BLOOD FLOW AND DEPRESSION

Nancy: In this section, Les is explaining the different factors that can affect blood flow.

The basic fact that is persistently ignored is that red blood cells come in a range of different shapes. The medical textbooks teach that all red blood cells are 'biconcave discocytes'. A biconcave discocyte is a cell (cyte) which is flat and round (disco) with a dimple (concave) on both sides (bi). These features combine to allow the cell to curl up and stretch out (deform) enough to slide easily through the tiny blood vessels (capillaries) that serve every cell in our body. The function of red blood cells is to carry oxygen to the cell and remove the waste products. Cells, and therefore the organs they serve, cannot function properly unless the red blood cells can reach them and do their job.

Les, and other researchers who study the physical properties of blood point out that red blood cells in fact come in a number of other shapes, which are clearly visible even in slides used to teach that all red blood cells are biconcave discocytes.

THE DETERMINANTS OF BLOOD FLOW

In order to appreciate the significance and implications of the many reports of reduced regional cerebral blood flow in depression, it is important that the reader is aware of those factors which may be involved in reducing the rate of cerebral blood flow.

Blood is a complex fluid and several factors determine how the blood flows. Such factors as whole blood viscosity, plasma viscosity and serum viscosity can provide useful information when measured. Red cell number is the major determinant of blood viscosity and when the haematocrit exceeds 0.48, it is likely that blood viscosity will be abnormally raised. When there is an increase in the blood of large molecules, such as fibrinogen, cholesterol, immunoglobulins and foreign proteins such as myeloma protein, an increased plasma viscosity will contribute to whole blood viscosity. On leaving the bone marrow, red cells lose their nucleus which renders them incapable of an independent existence, and they appear to be at the mercy of their environment. Changes in the internal environment which may follow both physiological stimuli, such as hormonal changes, or overexertion, or pathological stimuli, such as toxins or cancer, stimulate red cells to change to nondiscocytic forms; a change which is associated with reduced red cell deformability.

Nancy: Here Les is explaining that red blood cells may change their shape to a less deformable (flexible) one in response to a number of different changes in their environment. The important point is that if the cells change their shape to a less deformable one, they then cannot get through the capillaries, slowing down blood flow to areas especially where the capillaries are particularly small.

It needs to be recognised that the currently taught concept that all red cells are biconcave discocytes, is a consequence of red cells being exposed to anti-coagulants and washed in saline solutions prior to fixation, so the biconcave shape is a consequence of their processing.

> *Nancy: This important point offers some explanation for the continuing belief that all red blood cells are biconcave discocytes. The normal procedure with blood samples is to 'expose them to anti-coagulants' and wash them in saline solutions before being fixed for the purpose of being photographed. This process allows the shape-changed cells to revert to the biconcave discocyte shape. The range of shapes will only be seen in micrographs of 'immediately fixed' blood samples.*

Miller et al (29) in 1977, reported that red cells which had been taken directly into a fixative had different shapes from samples collected into anticoagulants. Others have reported similar findings and in 1989 Simpson (30) reported that the immediately fixed red cells of healthy humans and animals could be classified into six different shape classes, one of which was biconcave discocytes. In addition, there are several reports of changed red cell shapes in chronic disorders. For example, increased stomatocytes (cup forms) have been shown to occur in Huntington's Disease. (31) The relevant information has been summarised in a paper titled, "Red cell shape in health and disease." (32) A major problem is that writers of text books ignore those reports of shape-changed red cells. An example is, "An atlas of blood cells," by Zucker-Franklin et al, an authoritative reference text, which can be found in most haematology laboratories. (33) In volume 1, p 52, figure 2b is a micrograph of 39 red cells. The caption stated, *"By scanning electron microscopy, red cells appear as biconcave discocytes,"* but only 5 or 6 cells show that form.

The remaining 33 cells are flat, ridged or dimpled, and such forms are simply disregarded. **It is unclear why haematologists should continue with the pretence that all red cells are biconcave discocytes. The failure to recognise that nondiscocytic cells are less deformable than discocytes, means a lack of acceptance of the fact that an increase in the proportions of nondiscocytes, because of their reduced deformability, is not a benign event.**

> *Nancy:* *This last sentence, understated as it is, provides the whole explanation for the failure of modern medical practice to make use of relatively simple measures which could improve the lives of people suffering from depression, as well as many other chronic illnesses. Haematologists do not accept that red blood cells occur in a number of non-deformable—rigid—shapes, which cannot travel easily through the capillaries, so can interfere with oxygen delivery to specific cells, interfering with their ability to function normally. Therefore, situations in which these non-deformable cells occur in a higher proportion than usual are harmful—'not a benign event'.*

Red cell deformability is important because in the microcirculation, cells which are 7.5 to 8 microns in diameter must traverse capillary beds in which the mean capillary diameter is about 3.5 to 4 microns. When red cell deformability is reduced it is not unusual for plasma viscosity to be increased also, due to raised values of fibrinogen, cholesterol and/or immunoglobulins which will increase the resistance to flow.

There is little general appreciation of the fact that blood is a thixotropic system, in which its viscosity is determined by the rate of flow. In the major vessels where the flow rate is fast, blood viscosity is minimal, but when the rate of flow declines, blood viscosity increases. Professor John Dormandy (34) noted that," *This creates the apparent paradox that when the blood moves slowly it needs proportionately more driving force than when it moves fast.*" This means that if there is a slowing or cessation of blood flow, the resistance to flow will be increased because of the rise of blood viscosity. This change could be styled as thixotropic amplification of blood viscosity.

Because capillaries are the only channels through which oxygen and nutrient substrates are delivered to the tissues and waste metabolites are removed, normal tissue function is absolutely reliant on normal rates of capillary blood flow.

In his 1892 textbook on physiology, the father of British physiology, Professor Earnest Starling proposed that capillaries should be recognised as the chief part of the circulation. Arteries and veins were considered simply as the conduits which conveyed blood from and to the pump (the heart).

According to the Poiseuille formula, the rate of flow through narrow tubes is related directly to the fourth power of the tube radius. Fishberg (35) noted, *"While the laws of Poiseuille do not hold exactly for the branching circulation, it seems clear from the studies of Hess, Tigerstedt and others that they furnish valuable approximations which are at least of the correct order."* What is clear is that even very small reductions in vessel diameter lead to marked reductions in flow volume.

There are many observations which appear to indicate that throughout the body there are randomly distributed clusters of smaller than usual capillaries, which will become apparent in the presence of poorly deformable red cells. Furthermore, it is possible that a small proportion of the population will have smaller than usual mean capillary diameters. Such people may become dysfunctional after exposure to any agent which induces changes in cell shape and reduced red cell deformability. In 1992 (36) it was proposed that, *"Subjects with the symptom of tiredness and high percentages of nondiscocytic red cells in their blood would have smaller than usual capillaries; i.e. those with a mean capillary diameter falling within the first quartile of a capillary size distribution.* Such a concept of localised, smaller than usual capillaries, would provide an explanation for the reduced cerebral blood flow which has been recorded in the frontal regions of the brain of patients with depression.

> *Nancy:* *This observation—a random occurrence of smaller than usual capillaries—raises the interesting possibility that, if capillary size is relative to body size overall, this could provide a novel explanation for the proportionally higher incidence of both depression and other chronic illnesses in women. (Nothing to do with 'being hysterical'!).*

CEREBRAL BLOOD FLOW AND DEPRESSION

Since about 1965 there have been several hundreds of published reports relating to regional cerebral blood flow and depression. No attempt will be made to summarise all the available information. Instead, reference will be made to papers which exemplify the changes in cerebral blood flow which occur during depression. Up until about 1986, 133Xenon-based techniques were used, but since that time single photon emission computed tomography (SPET, SPECT) has been the most frequently used technique. An interesting feature of these findings is that there is a small group of studies the results from which differ from those of the majority. For example, in an American study in 1993 of 43 unipolar depressed subjects and 12 normal controls (37) it was noted, *"There were no significant differences in the distribution of Tc-99m-HMPAO into total regions of interest, right or left global regions of interest, pre-frontal, motor frontal, parietal, visual cortex or associative visual cortex between patients with melancholic depression, simple major depression or minor depression and healthy control subjects.*" The authors stated, "*It is concluded that cortical CBF as assessed with Tc-99m-HMPAO SPECT is relatively intact in the present sample of patients with severe depression.*" However, such observations conflict with a great many papers from Japan, Turkey, the USA, Poland, Slovenia and Germany which have reported reduced rates of regional cerebral blood flow during depression, but returned to normal during the remitted state. But it should be noted that there were variations in the sites in the brain which expressed reduced regional cerebral blood flow. Typical of such results is the English translation of the abstract of a paper in German (38) which noted that, "*At baseline all patients showed hypoperfusion in the left prefrontal cortex when compared with the right side,*" and the hypoperfusion was reversible on remission. There is a good deal of variation in the observations concerning left side/right side perfusion, and in the number of reports concerning changes in the cingulate cortex. A rather surprising aspect of such reports is the lack of discussion about the implications of the observed normalisation of blood flow in the remitted state. Dysfunction accompanied reductions in regional cerebral blood flow and normal function returned with the normalisation of blood flow. This raises the possibility that the dysfunction was a consequence of inadequate rates of delivery of oxygen and nutrient substrates to sustain normal tissue function. Such a situation, which involves a change from sub-normal to normal rates of blood flow, might best be explained in terms of changes in the flow properties of the blood. Many factors have the ability to alter the internal environment and red cells respond to such changes by changing shape. Non-discocytic red cells are poorly deformable and will impair capillary blood flow, but this change will be reversed when the internal environment returns to normal. Because poorly deformable red cells will have the greatest adverse effect in tissues where there are randomly distributed clusters of small capillaries, then it is possible that depression is a consequence of the presence of small capillaries in the left pre-frontal cortex. This proposal would be consistent with the findings of Lucey et al (39) who used SPET to study regional cerebral blood flow in patients suffering from obsessive compulsive disorder, panic disorder with agoraphobia or with post traumatic stress disorder. It was found that in all three disorders there were regions of reduced blood flow, but the regions with reduced blood flow were different in each disorder.

If changes in blood rheology are crucial factors in the development of depressive illness, then more frequent occurrence of depressive illness could be expected to occur in conditions known to have altered blood rheology such as poorly filterable blood, reduced red cell deformability and increased blood viscosity. Such changes are factors in aging, diabetes, cardiac disease and cerebrovascular disorders. If this is the case, then depressive illness in adolescents should show differences from depression in the elderly. In a Turkish study of adolescents with MDD (40) it was noted, "...*that adolescent patients with MDD may have regional cerebral blood flow deficits in frontal regions and a greater antero-frontal right-left perfusion asymmetry compared with normal subjects.*" An American study (41) found that, "*Adolescents with MDD show rCBF abnormalities similar to those found in adult MDD rCBF studies.*" But as noted previously, the blood of people older than about 55 years is more viscous and the red cells are stiffer than in younger people. According to Ishikawa et al (42), "*... in late-life depression there is little evidence of a longitudinal change in rCBF through remission.*" In 25 depressed patients older than 55 years, regional cerebral blood flow (rCBF) was reduced in the anterior ventral and dorsal medial prefrontal cortex. After pharmacotherapy, rCBF significantly increased in the left dorso-lateral prefrontal cortex and in other regions. " *However, decreased rCBF at baseline in the anterior ventral/dorsal medial prefrontal cortex, bilateral ventrolateral prefrontal cortex, bilateral temporal lobes and bilateral parietal lobes did not show significant improvement after treatment.*" Because the age-related changes in blood rheology appeared not to be known, such changes in blood flow were considered to be reflecting, "...*underlying and continuous pathognomonic brain dysfunction of depression (trait dependent).*" This conclusion would be compatible with the possibility that the pathognomonic factor was an interaction of smaller than usual capillaries with poorly deformable red cells.

Others have reported similar findings concerning cerebral blood flow in those responding to drug therapy as noted earlier. (35). Ogura et al (43) studied rCBF in 16 MDD patients while in the depressed state and during remission. In the depressed state, they found, "...*significant reductions in tracer uptake in the left superior frontal, bilateral parietal and right lateral temporal cortex.*" During remission, increased uptake occurred in all of these regions.

There are many reports which show that patients with refractory depression who respond to electroconvulsive therapy (ECT) have improved blood flow, although the mechanism involved with the increased blood flow is not discussed. Milo et al (44) reported the effects of ECT on 15 patients with MDD. They noted that prior to ECT, the patients exhibited hypoperfusion of the frontal regions, compared with controls. Only five patients had an excellent response to ECT and they exhibited changes towards normal rCBF. Non-responders, "...*showed no significant changes in rCBF.*" In a similar study (45) it was stated, "*Improvement in frontal and temporal hypoperfusion was seen only in those patients who responded to ECT.*" In a comparison of the benefits of drug therapy with ECT, Navarro et al (46) concluded, *"The long-term evolution of frontal perfusion in elderly major depressives who respond to antidepressant biological treatment is essentially the same in those who receive electroconvulsive therapy and in those who receive medication."* According to a PubMed search for "rTMS and depression" there have been 457 relevant studies of repetitive transcranial magnetic stimulation (rTMS) published since 1995. In the early studies the effects of the treatment were assessed by the extent of change in the Hamilton Depression score. Daily, left frontal rTMS was given to six medication-resistant depressed patients. (47) On the whole, the depression scores improved significantly and it was stated, *" Two subjects showed robust mood improvement which occurred progressively over several weeks. In one subject depression symptoms completely remitted for the first time in 3 years."* However, there were contrary findings in an Australian study (48) which concluded that, *"Repetitive transcranial magnetic stimulation did not provide significantly greater improvement than did sham treatment."* When the clinical effectiveness and cost effectiveness of ECT was compared with that of a 15 day course of rTMS over the left dorsolateral prefrontal cortex (49) it was concluded that ECT was a more cost effective treatment than 15 days of rTMS.

Between 2000 and 2007, ten papers which dealt with the effects of rTMS on cerebral blood flow, were published. Speer et al (50) studied the effects of both high and low frequency rTMS in 10 adults with MDD. They concluded, *"These data indicate that 2 weeks of daily 20-Hz rTMS over the left prefrontal cortex at 100%MT induce persistent increases in rCBF in bilateral frontal, limbic and paralimbic regions implicated in depression, whereas 1-Hz rTMS produced more circumscribed decreases."* Several other studies reported similar findings.

What is surprising is that although three different modes of treatment for MDD shared the common feature of improving rCBF, there was no discussion of what factor or factors might have been responsible for improving blood flow. Therefore, it is possible that the beneficial effects of psychotherapy could be due to the effects of counselling in lowering the stress levels which would result in improved capillary blood flow as the stress hormones have been shown to reduce blood filterability.

There is a major lack of information concerning the physical properties of the blood in people when they are suffering from depression, and during remission. An inability to obtain the co-operation of psychologists and psychiatrists means that I have no data about blood filterability, (a measure of red cell deformability) blood viscometry and red cell shape changes in people during an episode of depression or in remission. But in chapter 7 of his 1976 book (51) Dintenfass had sections on "Stress" and "Senility, depression and other mental conditions." In the section on stress, he noted that there were several papers which reported that emotional factors resulted in, *"An elevation of capillary resistance and blood pressure."* He quoted a 1967 paper in which the author, *"…was able to predict successfully, sudden death among coronary patients on the basis of depression, long-term frustration in jobs or in a family setting"* all of which were stressful factors. Later he stated, *"The viscosity of blood was observed to be elevated in the emotional stress evoked by depression, worries or 'bad news'."* So the occurrence of increased blood viscosity in depression has been known for a long time. In the section on Senility etc, he included the findings of a study involving 632 mentally defective patients and 115 patients with Down's syndrome. Plasma viscosity was 5% to 20% higher in the patients than in controls. On the basis of the findings of others which proposed that pre-senile dementia was a result of *"arterial insufficiency,"* he noted that senile and pre-senile dementia could be prevented by anticoagulant therapy with dicoumarol. This led him to state, "...*thus substantiating the fact that mental disorders might be a direct result of occlusive circulatory disorders.*" In a series of papers he showed that patients suffering from depressive or schizoid anxiety were different from normals in terms of blood viscosity and in some biochemical factors. Patients with chronic anxiety had significantly higher plasma and blood viscosity. It was stated:

> "*The general level of abnormalities of blood viscosity factors (plasma and blood viscosity, aggregation of red cells, apparent viscosity of artificial thrombi) could suggest that depressive and schizoid anxiety patients (in particular the depressive anxiety patients) show a concurrent pathorheology of blood flow and coagulation.*"

It would appear that Dintenfass was unaware of a 1975 paper by Rasmussen et al (52) which reported that the stress hormones reduced the filterability of blood (presumably by reducing the deformability of the red cells), but he stated, "*It is not possible yet to state whether anxiety is the cause or the result of an elevation of blood viscosity. But by its very presence an elevation of blood viscosity might affect the cardiovascular or cerebral circulation, and it might form a link between anxiety and vascular disorders. The question would be whether a release of anxiety by any means will lead to a decrease of blood viscosity or any of the blood viscosity factors.*" In a continuation of this line of thought concerning the relationship between physical and psychological illnesses, he stated, "*One could wonder also whether a treatment of the psychological (mental) illness should not, or could not, include a modification of the blood viscosity factors. At least in one example of senility (pre-senile dementia) a decrease of blood viscosity appears to be beneficial.*"

Do the mechanisms of Alzheimer's disease provide useful information about depression?

The absence of any information about red cell shape changes during depression is a basic problem when the objective is to show that depression is primarily a problem of blood flow. However, Alzheimer's disease is an age-related disorder in which depression may develop, and there is a good deal of published information about the aging process, blood flow and the physical properties of the blood. A Swedish study (25) of cerebral blood flow in 97 healthy subjects aged between 19 and 68 years concluded that,"...*the mean cerebral blood flow decreases progressively with age.*" A similar conclusion was reached in a British study (51) of regional cerebral blood flow in 30 normal volunteers aged between 30 and 80 years. The authors concluded, *"Decrease in regional cerebral blood flow suggest a regionally specific loss of cerebral function with age."* Ajmani and Rifkind (28) reported in 1998 that the aging process was accompanied by a rise in plasma levels of fibrinogen, together with increases in whole blood viscosity, plasma viscosity and red cell rigidity. More recently, Carallo et al (54) assessed the effects of aging on blood rheology factors in blood samples taken 11.6 years apart. Although it was concluded that, *"The present findings demonstrate that blood viscosity increases with age,"* and that red cell rigidity increased with age, they did not relate such changes to any other factor. So it could be important that in 1972, Cerny et al (24) had reported that blood viscosity was much higher in older people than in the young. They noted that , *"The tendency for blood viscosity to be greater at low shear rate, probably reflected the presence of poorly deformable red cells."* In 2003, Simpson and O'Neill (55) showed the age-related changes in red cell shape which occurred between 60 and 96 years of age. This means that in the age group which develops Alzheimer's disease, blood viscosity increases would be accompanied by the presence of shape-changed, poorly deformable red cells. Such observations are similar to those recorded in 1986 when people suffering from myalgic encephalomyelitis (ME), a condition in which depression may be a problem, were shown to have poorly filterable blood. (56) Later, (57) it was shown that symptomatic ME sufferers were shown to have shape-changed, red cells which would account for the reduced filterability.

Such observations make it reasonable to propose that the increased blood viscosity in depression is accompanied by shape-changed, poorly deformable red cells, which would play a significant role in determining the rate of rCBF in depression. This would be consistent with the observation that those who respond to treatments have improved blood flow, as this implies that during depression rCBF is in some way reduced. A reasonable guess to explain the observations is that in some unexplained manner the treatments normalise the internal environment, thus enabling red cells to assume their usual shapes with normal levels of red cell deformability, thus improving capillary blood flow. As no published report concerning the physical properties of the blood in depressed subjects has been located, it seems reasonable to conclude that the depression which occurs in patients with Alzheimer's disease is related to changes in the physical properties of the blood and in red cell shape.

> **Nancy:** *Les here explains that because he was unable to obtain the cooperation of psychiatrists for his research, he was unable to obtain blood samples from depressed patients. He therefore has to rely on the reports of other researchers concerning the effect of emotional stress on blood viscosity. He also speculates that the depression which occurs with Alzheimer's may be due to known changes in blood viscosity in older people.*

NANCY, AGAIN:
SO WHAT ABOUT THIS INTERNAL DIALOGUE?

The previous section has elaborated at several points how psychotherapy, by reducing stress, can be a factor in improving blood flow. Now that we have a physiological explanation of how psychotherapy helps, it is time to return to how it is done.

Often self-help books suggest that we listen to our self-critical voice, hear the words and sentences, and then substitute positive 'affirmations'. Look in the mirror and tell ourselves that we are attractive, accomplished, good people. The problem is that we don't actually believe these things (even if they happen to be true! And, you know what, they probably *are* true….).

The first step in working with internal dialogue is to begin to notice it. Although most of you will know exactly what I mean, we are not always in the habit of paying conscious attention to it. Rather, it seems to play itself, a dismal verbal Muzak to our everyday lives. It's a novel concept that we can begin to edit our own backing track! It can be instructive just to pay attention to the words that are being said, the criticisms that we are levelling at ourselves. We may notice that they are not in fact very accurate—but we may not. We are very accustomed to believing this annoying little voice.

Once we allow ourselves to focus on this internal voice, we can begin to ask ourselves questions about it. Whose voice is it? Is it the voice of a parent, or of some other important individual in our lives? Is it our own voice? Where does it seem to be coming from? Behind us? From the right? The left? Is it 'all around' ?

We've always just taken it for granted, and suffered the feelings that it engenders in us, just as though there were some other person standing there, uttering a stream of critical comments. As we begin to notice the voice itself, we may begin to wonder about the words it is saying. Let's pay some more attention to that later, but in the meantime, pretend it is a voice coming out of a radio. Or your earphones. Can you turn the radio down, or off; can you put your earphones down, or change the channel, or get a different player that has a different sound-track?

If we imagine it coming out of a radio, we can move it around. If the radio seems to be on our left, let's see what happens when we move it around to the right. If it seems to be playing behind us, what happens when we put it in front of us, instead?

As you experiment with moving its location, notice how moving it around changes it in other ways. Maybe it is harder to hear when it's on the right. Maybe when it's in front instead of behind, the words tend to change. Maybe it gets louder, and we want to move it back again. In certain locations, the words may affect us more strongly. In other locations, it may seem unimportant, just a trivial background noise. In doing this, you are discovering that you can take control of some of your mental processes, and that when you change your sense of the location of the voice, you can also change how it affects you. Now you have some choice.

(And at this point, you will notice in yourself what a psychotherapist might call 'resistance'. You don't even want to

feel better. Feeling better would somehow be uncomfortable, not right. You are used to feeling terrible, feeling better is unfamiliar, a bit unnerving, just wrong! It feels safer just to keep the radio where you hear it and feel it the most.)

So this is the time to introduce you to an important presupposition of NLP—*There is no such thing as failure, only feedback.* If you find it difficult, or impossible, to follow the instructions above, this is nothing more than than an invitation to learn more about your mental processing by examining what is getting in the way—or to explore other options — and there are lots of other options.

We have considered the location of the inner dialogue. There are lots of other features of any sound, or voice. There is the volume—it is loud or soft? Can you make it louder? Can you turn the volume down? If you can, you will notice which volume has the most, and the least, emotional effect on you. Making the voice louder may make it more forceful and frightening. Imagining it being bellowed out on the stage of an opera might make it even worse—or it might make it begin to seem ridiculous. (If we are in a therapy session, playing with these changes, and you start to smile, or even giggle, we know that's a change you want to keep going!). Sometimes turning the volume down makes the emotional effect fade. For some of us, a whisper might seem even more sinister and threatening. (Or, to use the operatic analogy—it could become the exaggerated whisper in one of those old black-and-white film melodramas that look so silly.) The point is that you are the expert on what works for you—you are free to experiment and make your own discoveries. Once you know how to change it so that the emotional effect changes, you are in control.

There is one kind of change that I particularly enjoy teaching to my clients: the speed. Some of us are old enough to remember the jolt produced when you put your favourite 33rpm record on the player, and the speed was set at 78! For those of you who have never had this experience, it turns the most profoundly emotional symphony or opera into a series of high-pitched squeaks. Taking that serious, forbidding inner voice and speeding it up first turns it into Mickey Mouse, then as it gets faster and faster, more and more high-pitched, it turns into a tinny whine, just before it reaches the frequencies we can't even hear any more—the frequency of a 'silent' dog whistle, or the squeaks audible only to bats as they echolocate around the cave. Just think what it would be like to practice speeding the voice up like this, every time it started, until your brain simply did it automatically! The 'space' that would be created, for you to have other feelings, other thoughts....to reclaim the energy this voice had taken away from you....worth a try?

And here is one for all of you who struggle, especially when trying to go to sleep, or lying awake in the early morning—when your thoughts go round and round, and you just wish you had a way to switch them off. As you are telling me about your thoughts going 'round and round', you are likely to make a circle with your hand to demonstrate this. Try this out—try to find the gesture. If you can make this gesture, notice which way your hand is going. Just allow the circling to continue while you figure this out. When you have figured it out, then reverse it—move your hand in a circle in the opposite direction. This takes concentration, and as you do so, you will find that the thought patterns simply break up. This happens because our whole system is linked—our thoughts, our feelings, our posture, our breathing, our physical movements. So here is another way that you can break up the patterns of thought that are part of depression. You wanted to find some way to stop that endless circling—and this may be that way. This is just another deceptively effective technique that is so simple that it sounds silly, and if doing it makes you laugh…so much the better!

To recap: Once you have experienced how the depression process is linked to looking down, listening to your self-critical internal dialogue, and feeling bad, here are several strategies you can experiment with. It has probably never occurred to you before that you could actually take charge of your thought processes, (your *'subjective experience'*—how you feel in your life) and make deliberate choices about them. You don't have to be the passenger in the ride your mind takes you on— you can become the driver. You can even become the engineer who can look under the bonnet, and make a couple of apparently minor changes that will improve how the whole things works! Bandler would tell you not to bother about whether these things are 'true' or not. A set of instructions is just a set of instructions—follow them carefully, and if you get the outcome you want—use them. If you've followed them carefully and you don't get the outcome you want—you're free to throw them away! But make sure that you did follow them carefully....

Now let's move on to more ways that we can begin to shift and shape the mental/emotional activities which up to now haven't allowed us to feel good about ourselves, to enjoy our lives.

VICTIM GUILT

The phenomenon of 'victim guilt', in people who have suffered extreme degrees of abuse or punishment, can be one of the most difficult aspects for a therapist to try to change. To an outsider, it seems obvious that a child (or an adult) being mistreated in some way would feel anger towards the perpetrator, and that the perpetrator is the one who should feel guilty. What is the mechanism by which this gets so badly confused? Victims of abuse, rape, domestic violence, so often feel, not angry at the perpetrator, but rather, ashamed and guilty. (Often, the family system goes along with this - the victim who complains is accused of damaging the family, as though the perpetrator is doing no wrong, the only wrong lies in exposing it. We are horrified by cultures in which female victims of rape are condemned to death for adultery, but too often in our own judicial system, the victim's dress—skirt too short, behaviour—she was drunk - or past history, become grounds for dismissing her claim of rape—'she was asking for it'.)

So there are cultural pressures which encourage victims to blame themselves—it wasn't that long ago when having cancer was treated as a shameful secret, and today we are encouraged to see disability as a self-serving myth, and poverty and unemployment as a result of moral failings rather than symptoms of economic injustice or genuine misfortune. Poverty, injustice, misfortune are all realistic reasons to feel depressed. Helplessness, lack of control over ones situation, is linked to depression. The labelling of depression as a medical problem can serve a political purpose by directing attention away from the policies which create the conditions that result in hardship. Convincing people that their poverty, unemployment or disability are their own fault[7] is a

---

[7] An extreme example of this is the treatment of people who suffer from ME/CFS, a disabling, multi-symptom autoimmune disorder which is defined by the fact that muscular and/or cognitive effort has a delayed and protracted effect, making all the symptoms worse. Severely ill patients are unable to perform even slight activities and are in unremitting pain and hypersensitivity, often for years. Insistence that this is a psychiatric disorder is used to justify incarceration of adults, removal of sick children from their parents care, and subjection to exercise regimes and psychological and physical abuse, for example leaving food out of reach. When patients become worse under this treatment, they are labelled 'treatment resistant'. Even recorded deaths from this illness fail to make any impact on the prevailing view that this is something patients are choosing to do to themselves.

cultural/political way of creating 'victim guilt'. One way to resist depression is to study the causes of these situations, decline to feel guilty, and seek out some form of action to address these issues.

We can see that 'victim guilt' can be used for political ends, and is also used too often in the way that victims of sexual violence are treated. But how does our vulnerability to victim guilt arise in the first place?

Consider the human infant. We are born entirely helpless, entirely dependent on the willingness of someone around us to respond to our cries, and meet our needs.

Our culture is rather contemptuous of 'attention-seeking behaviour'. (How often do we hear 'she/he's only doing it for attention'.) But—consider this: **From the moment we are born, our physical survival depends completely on our being able to 'get attention'.** The frantic screaming of the hungry baby tells us the infant senses that getting attention is truly a matter of life or death. Unless there is another person present who has both the knowledge and the power to provide the things we need, and who loves us enough to 'pay attention', we **are** going to die.

This is the basis of our instinctive objection to child-rearing practices which involve protracted periods of failure to respond to a child's crying, or even practicing a principle of not responding. A caretaker who pays attention, who reassures the child that his cries will bring the adult to him, is teaching the child to feel safe in the world, to create the beginnings of a sense of self-worth, of being lovable. The adult who is paying attention will learn what different cries mean—whether the child is hungry, in discomfort or pain, tired, or just bad-tempered. The child who feels safe in the world can tolerate delays in having his needs met; comforted and loved, then left to go to sleep, his tired crying will soon fade into a peaceful sleep. A child whose cries get no response will progress from terrified and hysterical weeping into the passivity of despair. Not the same thing.

Very early in life, we begin to learn that certain things please our caretakers, and certain things displease them. If we are fortunate, those who look after us will find us lovable—we will learn from them that we are a source of joy and pride, although there will be times when we will find that we displease them; that there are rules to be learned and followed.

If we are not so fortunate, if we suffer neglect or abuse, we learn to experience ourselves very differently. There is little we can do to please our caretakers. But as infants and small children, we cannot conceptualise adults being anything other than perfect beings—otherwise we are utterly endangered. If those around us don't have the knowledge required to meet our needs, and the power in the world that is needed to provide for us, or don't love us enough to bother, we are in mortal danger. It is safer to believe that it is we who are at fault, because then we can imagine that if we can find a way to 'be good', our needs will be met. Therefore children who grow up with parents who are themselves depressed, or ill, or at odds with each other are very likely to feel—to want to believe —that whatever it is, is their fault. *Because if it is their fault, then maybe they can make it better, by trying harder to be good. (And if they fail, it must mean they are not good enough.)*

In that scenario, the seeds of depression are sown.

This is why it is important for parents in difficult circumstances to try to find ways to explain to children what is going on. Left to themselves, they will wonder whether 'it's anything I've done'. Rather than try to keep secrets, or 'protect' children from unhappy truths, we need to try to help them understand what is going on. Otherwise we are laying the ground for the typical depressive tendency to feel guilty and responsible for events which realistically are out of our control.

If bad things happen, and are not explained, or needed things are not provided, the safest conclusion to reach is that we must deserve it. Believing that bad things happen because of the way that we are, at least creates the illusion that if we can find some way to 'be good', things will be better. It is the only way to imagine that we have some power in the situation. Painful as it is, to assume that the bad events that occur are our fault is the least frightening option.

This isn't just a tendency in individuals. As mentioned above, history includes many tales of natural disasters which were interpreted as 'the wrath of the gods', punishments for sins of the whole population.

I believe that it is this—the illusion of power created by a belief that bad events must be 'our fault', therefore that if we can figure out how to be good, (how to appease the gods!) the bad events will stop—which lays the foundation for 'victim guilt', and makes it so difficult to relinquish.

How does NLP offer us ways to resolve this?

SUBMODALITIES

We have already covered the subject of *representational systems*, and *sequences* of mental behaviour. When we learn that depression is operated through looking down (external visual), listening to our inner critical voice - (internal, Internal Dialogue), and feeling sad/guilty (Internal, kinaesthetic), we are looking at a *sequence* of mental behaviour. When we replace the first step in the depression sequence with looking up (visual external), we find that we no longer have access to the further steps in the depression sequence. This effect is enhanced if we have also changed our slumped physical position to sitting or standing in an erect posture, and if we engage in physical activity (the kinesthetics of actual physical movement). (Linking to what Les has to tell us, physical movement will in itself improve blood flow, which will have a positive physical effect on what is happening in our brain.)

In addition, we have experimented with the 'submodalities' of our internal dialogue. When we were considering our inner self-critical voice, we discussed changing its location, its volume, and its speed. All of these are 'auditory submodalities'.

In visual representations, the power of changed submodalities can be illustrated by some simple examples. For those of us of an older generation, who may have been subjected to (sorry, surely I meant 'enjoyed'!) slide shows of other people's holidays, there is a major difference between the effect of the images on a set of photos handed round, or slide projected on a big screen. Film theatres use this to the maximum—we experience the combined effect of images on a huge screen and very loud sounds, projected all around us. Size, clarity of image, bright realistic colour, the volume and realistic quality of sound produce the most powerful emotional impact, as well as a sense of being in the experience, not just watching it.

Now think about the way you mentally represent your past experiences. A major part of the way our brain functions has the purpose of keeping us alive. (In fact one could say that every bit of how our organism functions has the purpose of keeping us alive—which opens the concept of having to fight against, or control, 'bad' aspects of ourselves, to re-consideration.) If there is danger in a particular environment, or a particular activity, there is a part of our brain dedicated to producing an immediate response—fight or flight—happening much more quickly than our conscious awareness can kick in. If you are a driver, you can probably remember times when you have found yourself reaching for the brakes a split second before you realised what the hazard was that you were responding to. As life goes on, we form more and more conscious and unconscious links to places, events, people, associated with threats to our well-being; this is why we tend to have more vivid, emotionally powerful memories of negative events than our happier ones. Our survival doesn't depend on remembering, associating to and responding emotionally to situations in which we were happy and safe, so these memories tend to have less impact. But clearly, if our life experiences have predominantly been negative or traumatic, we are likely to have quite an overload of these protective reactions.

When we remember traumatic events, it is most likely that we *relive* them, experience the negative emotions we experienced at the time, reinforcing whatever bad time we are having in the present. Unfortunately, most forms of psychotherapy encourage us to do this, from a belief that somehow this re-living of the experience will gradually reduce its impact on us. But the more we are encouraged to re-live it, as accurately as possible, the more the negative emotions and beliefs formed at the time will be reinforced. This is why psychotherapy is usually experienced as traumatic in itself, something expected to be painful and difficult. And expected to take a long time. And, sadly, often unhelpful.

Cognitive Behaviour Therapy, (as well as the Egan model often taught in counselling courses) by contrast, endeavours to make use only of your capacity for conscious, rational thought, thus constraining its impact because it fails to make use of the strengths and resources residing outside our limited ability to manage our behaviour through logical reasoning. 'Don't be silly, dear' is not generally a helpful admonition. If common sense could solve our problem, we wouldn't need to ask for anyone's help.

In NLP, we use the term 'associated' to refer to experiencing a memory as though we are reliving it. In the case of traumatic memories, we encourage our clients to 'dissociate'—to remain aware that they are now in the present time, in a safe situation—while 're-viewing' the memory. This means to be looking at it as though it had been filmed at the time, or videoed, and we are now watching the event—seeing ourselves as one of the actors, judging the experience that that person is having, from the perspective of an outside observer.

An example of how this works is a very depressed young woman who had been gang-raped outside her secondary school when she was younger. A friend who had been with her when these youths accosted them had escaped by running away immediately. She had not run away, and firmly believed that that made her to blame for what had then happened. This self-blame had continued to contaminate her life, and she was at the point of contemplating suicide. When, in the therapeutic situation, we finally had created a sense of safety in which she was able to watch this event, as though from a distance, framed as a scene in a TV drama viewed on a small screen, she was able to see that what had kept her there was the fact that one of the youths had grabbed her purse—which contained money that had been entrusted to her by her grandmother, to bring in her week's shopping. Coming from a very poor background, she could not contemplate going home without this money, and she had tried to get her purse back. Seeing that in fact there had been a very good reason for her failure to escape, she was able to re-evaluate the whole situation. This was the beginning of a gradual recovery of her own self-respect.

In another example, a client who had a phobia of water came to me because he needed to pass a test connected with his profession which required him to learn underwater rescue skills. He recalled having been thrown into water by a swimming instructor dismissive of his initial timidity, when he was only six. He nearly drowned, had to be rescued, to the contempt of the instructor and the laughter of the rest of the children, and his embarrassed parents were told to take him home. What he 'learned' at the time was that water was dangerous, that he couldn't swim, and that he was therefore a laughing stock and a failure, as well as an embarrassment to his family. It was hardly surprising that this had developed into a full-blown phobia.

Helped to 'review' this situation, from the perspective of the competent adult and parent he had become, he now experienced, not the terror and shame of the child, but the anger of a parent seeing a child so mistreated. Further NLP techniques in this kind of situation involve inviting the client to imagine going into the scene, with whatever powers they need to deal with it, giving the child the comfort and support the child needed within the situation, and dealing appropriately with the adult involved. (Possibly getting him sacked!)

To objections that one cannot change the past, the reply is that that is true—but what is causing the current emotional distress is that that event has been recorded in our brain in a particular way. We can change the way that the event is recorded, therefore change its emotional impact. **In fact, a memory which has been recoded in this way has not been falsified, it has been corrected:** the facts of the matter in the first case are that the young girl had behaved with courage trying to do the right thing, and the subsequent events were the criminal behaviour of a gang of young men. In the second case, the facts were that a worried child perfectly able to learn to swim was mistreated by an incompetent and bullying adult. The technique of 're-viewing' past memories allows us to change the emotional impact of memories which up to then have contributed to the self criticism and guilt characteristic of depression, and this involves correcting the misunderstandings created at the time.

Using this means of 'recoding' a memory, in the part of our brain where it is stored, will mean that at least part of our depressive thought patterns, feelings, and ongoing self criticism will be undermined and altered at source. We can't change what happened, but we can change what we think and how we feel about what happened.

Using this process when our childhood experiences were of ongoing situations in which we felt inappropriately responsible, inadequate or to blame is a lengthy and more complicated process, but the principles are the same. The mother who doesn't respond to her infant because of her own illness or depression, family conflicts in which a child is a helpless witness, parental struggles with material deprivation, or with specific misfortunes, all can lead an infant or young child to feel bad about themselves and sow the seeds of adult depression.

When such events are recalled more accurately as due to external factors, and one can begin to see the child one was as an innocent and well-intentioned but relatively helpless part of the family drama, then the self-criticism and guilt typical of depression can begin to be drained away.

BACK TO LES:
TREATMENT OF THE BLOOD FLOW PROBLEMS OF PATIENTS WITH DEPRESSION

Even though blood flow returns to normal during remissions, there are several options for improving the flow properties of the blood in those who suffer from depression. All such agents could have particular significance for the elderly suffering from depression, which could be due in part to their age-related, increased blood viscosity.

(a) Changes in lifestyle.

As there is a substantial literature which documents the adverse effects of smoking on blood viscosity and red cell deformability, it is important that those who suffer from depression should cease to smoke cigarettes. Several studies have shown that after three weeks of cessation from smoking, the flow properties of the blood return to normal. Although it has been shown that those suffering from depression who responded to drug therapy or to electroconvulsive therapy or repetitive transcranial magnetic stimulation, had improved blood flow, the mechanism remains unexplained. No studies which dealt with the consequences of improved blood flow in depressed people were located. However, the results of studies of treatment of coronary heart disease by dietary changes could be informative. Dietary changes may be helpful, particularly if the current diet is high in saturated fats and accompanied by a raised level of cholesterol, and low fat diets have been shown to be helpful in different disorders. Low-fat diets with 10% or less of saturated fat, such as the Swank low-fat diet, have been shown to be an effective treatment for multiple sclerosis by improving bodily function and extending lifespan (58). In 1990, The Lancet published a report of a study in which heart disease patients were treated with dietary and lifestyle changes, without the use of drugs. (59) The fat content of the diet was restricted to the equivalent of 10% of total calories and excluded all animal products except for some skim milk and yoghurt. There was no restriction on plant-based foods which included vegetables, grains and fruit. Other lifestyle changes included meditation, relaxation and a regular exercise regimen. Maintenance of this lifestyle was accompanied by a fall in average levels of cholesterol from 227mg/dl to 172 mg/dl and with a marked reduction in low density lipoprotein. There was a marked reduction in all aspects of chest pains. Esselstyn et al (60) investigated the effects of a plant-based diet in people with established heart disease, with the objective of lowering the patients' blood cholesterol level to 150mg/dl. Participants in the study were not permitted to have meat, fish, fowl, oils and dairy products. During the first five years of the study five participants dropped out. At the beginning of the study, the remaining eighteen participants had average blood cholesterol levels of 246mg/dl. During the study, not only did the "bad" low density lipoprotein cholesterol drop dramatically, but also the average cholesterol level fell to 132mg/dl. Seventeen of the participants had no heart problems during the following eleven years, while one, who strayed from the diet, had an episode of angina which resolved when he returned to the plant-based diet. As both studies showed similar benefits, it is of some significance that the 1990 study noted that in those who kept to their diet, there was a reduction in the size of the arterial blockages. This lesion reversibility draws attention to a 1958 report, which showed that the inner layers of the human aorta (the media and intima) are not supplied with blood from the capillary network of the vasa vasorum. (61) On p 360 it was noted, *"There are no capillary vessels in the tunica media of normal arteries,"* and *"...nutrition of the intima and inner part of the media is maintained by filtration of nutrients from the arterial lumen."* Of particular significance is the statement: *"As filtration occurs at the pressure of arterial blood, fluid probably enters the intima from the lumen at a relatively high rate, yet any colloidal constituents, the proteins and lipoproteins which are normally returned to the blood via the lymph, have to diffuse across a broad avascular zone and through several laminae of elastic tissue before reaching the nearest lymphatics."* Later it was stated, *"There is also evidence that an increase in the arterial blood pressure predisposes to atherosclerosis. This association is seen not only in generalised hypertension, but also when the rise in tension is localised, etc."*

In general, endothelial cells will inhibit filtration from the blood stream, as they shield the basement membrane. Conversely, the most permeable microvessels, such as those in glomeruli have fenestrated endothelium. Simpson (62) has explained capillary permeability in terms of the thixotropic nature of basement membranes which have pressure-dependent permeability. Thus, the greater the intravascular pressure, the larger the molecules which are able to pass across the basement membrane. When considering the filtration across the arterial wall, it is noteworthy that the lipids in the intima are qualitatively the same as in the plasma. This implies that the basement membrane permits the passage of lipids at normal intravascular pressure. But when blood pressure is increased and there is a rise in cholesterol levels, more cholesterol than normal will pass into the intima and by its accumulation presents as an atherosclerotic lesion. As Ornish et al (59) reported that after a year on a low-fat diet, the size of the arterial blockages diminished, this could imply that the treatment not only lowered cholesterol levels but also blood pressure, thus reducing the rate of filtration into the atherosclerotic region. Subsequent diffusion to the lymphatics would reduce the volume of the lesion. Such a scenario would be consistent with the observation of Ornish et al.

> **Nancy:** *The advice to stop smoking and adopt a low-fat mainly vegetable-based diet seems sound, but not the easiest advice to follow!*

(b) The consequences of inactivity.

A study of the effects of bed rest on blood rheology, after total hip replacement, included observations on a control group of normal volunteers who were kept in bed for five days. (63) After five days of bed rest, blood tests from the control group showed an increase in haematocrit, a number of changes in blood chemistry which included an increase in fibrinogen, together with increases in blood and plasma viscosity. Such changes would have an adverse effect on the flow properties of the blood. A later paper titled, "Exercise and arthritis. The hematology of inactivity" (64) reported similar findings. It was stated, *"The hematology of inactivity comprises the following: low plasma volume, high hematocrit, high plasma fibrinogen, elevated blood viscosity, increased platelet aggregability and diminished fibrinolysis. Regular exercise reverses all these adverse blood changes and, thereby, helps prevent heart attack and stroke."* Such reports provide the factual background to studies dealing with the effects of exercise in patients with depression. Blumenthal et al (65) reported the effects of exercise training on older patients with major depression, which involved 156 subjects, 50 years of age or older who suffered from MDD. In a randomised, controlled study, participants were assigned to a programme of aerobic exercise;

medication (sertraline hydrochloride); or a combination of both exercise and medication for 16 weeks. It was concluded that, *"An exercise training programme may be considered as an alternative to anti-depressant treatment for depression in older persons..... after 16 weeks of treatment exercise was equally effective in reducing depression among patients with MDD."* In a later report concerning the same 156 volunteers (66) it was noted that after 10 months, the relapse rate was much lower for those in the exercise group than for those in the medication group. It was concluded, *" Among individuals with MDD, exercise therapy is feasible and is associated with significant therapeutic benefit, especially if exercise is continued over time."* Mather et al (67) investigated the effects of exercise on the depression of older adults who had responded poorly to treatment. They concluded, *" Because exercise was associated with a modest improvement in depressive symptoms at 10 weeks, older people with poorly responsive depressive disorder should be encouraged to attend group exercise activities."* The concept of "group exercise activities" was manifested in an Australian study in which women suffering from post-natal depression undertook exercise in the form of pram-pushing groups. (68) The authors noted:

> *"The results showed that mothers in the pram-walking intervention group improved their fitness levels and reduced their level of depressive symptomatology significantly more than the social support group."*

What is of some importance, is that none of the reports relating to the benefits of exercise for those suffering from depression made any reference to published studies concerning the effects of exercise on the flow properties of the blood. In 1987, Ernst published a paper titled, "Influence of regular physical activity on blood rheology." (69) He stated, *"This suggests that an improvement in blood fluidity can be induced by regular physical exercise, regardless of whether the blood rheology was normal or abnormal at baseline."* That observation was consistent with the changes in blood viscosity noted by others after bed rest (63) or after inactivity.(64) Such findings provide the link between blood viscosity-impaired blood flow and the manifestation of depressive illness. So there are good reasons to propose that those suffering from depression would benefit from undertaking a regular programme of physical activity, either in a group or as an individual.

> **Nancy:** *The advice to engage in exercise may be easier to follow – it is possible to build exercise into ones daily routine. However it is easy to underestimate the amount of physical exertion involved in housework and especially the care of young children. What depressed young mothers need probably includes more help and more company! From that perspective, group pram-walking makes sense. However in more recent times, young mothers are likely to join mother and toddler groups, which offer social contacts but not necessarily exercise.*

(c) The use of dietary supplements.

A feature of the reports dealing with the effects of exercise is that they draw attention to the role of raised blood viscosity in impairing blood flow. So it seems reasonable to suggest that agents which have been shown to lower blood viscosity could be useful in preventing the rise in blood viscosity which leads to the development of depressive illness. On the basis of published information, it seems that two such agents, namely extract of Gingko biloba and fish oil rich in omega-3 fatty acids, are worthy of discussion. There are many extracts of Gingko biloba available, but they are far from being homogeneous, while the most studied extract is a German product, EGb761. However, this lack of homogeneity is reflected in the high level of conflicting results. For example, Huang et al (70) reported that after three months of treatment with EGb761, patients with type 2 diabetes showed a significant reduction in blood viscosity and the deformability of red cells was increased by 20%. A consequence of such changes was improved retinal blood flow. While many studies report changes which would indicate a lowering of blood viscosity, many studies restrict their observations to plasma viscosity. However, two reports from the same group in Brazil reported that an undefined extract of Gingko biloba reduced blood viscosity. (71,72) Another study(73) assessed the effect of EGb761 on neuropsychologic functioning in older adults. The authors concluded that six weeks treatment with the extract, "...*may prove efficacious in enhancing certain neurocognitive functions/processes of cognitively intact older adults.*" A different extract (EGb Li 1370) was found to be effective, and it was noted, " *EGb significantly improved sleep pattern by an increase in sleep efficiency and a reduction in awakenings.*" It was suggested, "...*that the extract may provide a new treatment strategy especially in the treatment of the depressive syndrome with sleep disturbance.*" (74) Although a review of clinical studies in which EGb761 was used in the treatment of peripheral arterial occlusive disease concluded that, "*This review confirms the efficacy of Gingko biloba special extract EGb761,*" (75) it should be noted that there are many reports which claimed that Gingko biloba extracts were ineffective. A study of the effects of Gingko biloba extract PB246 showed that it failed to prevent the development of winter depression. (76) Similarly, in a Dutch study of the effects of EGb761 in elderly subjects with dementia and age-associated memory impairment (77) it was concluded, "*The results of our trial suggest that gingko is not effective as a treatment for older people with mild to moderate dementia or age-associated memory impairment. Our results contrast sharply with those of previous gingko trials.*" A study of the effects of a Gingko biloba extract of no stated origin, on patients with anti-depressant-induced sexual dysfunction (78) concluded that, "*This study did not replicate a prior positive finding supporting the use of Gingko biloba for anti-depressant, especially SSRI, induced sexual dysfunction.*" At this time it is not possible to provide a rational explanation for the frequent occurrence of conflicting results from the use of Gingko biloba extracts, although to some extent it may reflect variability in the nature of the extracts.

> ***Nancy:*** *This would suggest some cautious experimentation with Gingko biloba might be worth undertaking.*

(d) Fish oil.

Interest in the health aspects of the omega-3 fatty acids, eicosapentaenoic (EPA) and docsahexanoic (DHA) acids developed as a consequence of the rarity of heart disease among Eskimos and some American Indian tribes. Both races shared the common feature of having diets rich in fatty fish and animals. A brief report by a Japanese team in 1981 noted that EPA lowered blood viscosity. (79) A later report from the same group (80) stated that in healthy subjects EPA derived from sardine oil reduced blood viscosity and increased red blood cell deformability. The latter change reflected a marked increase in the phospholipid content of the erythrocyte membrane. Since that time others have reported similar findings. Harris et al (81) reported that after four weeks on a salmon oil supplement, there was a reduction in the plasma levels of both triglycerides and cholesterol. Another study (82) showed that fish oil taken as 10ml daily of MaxEPA, lowered blood viscosity in association with a significant reduction in triglycerides but without change in the levels of total cholesterol. However, when the dose of MaxEPA was increased to 16ml daily, the triglyceride levels were lowered by 58% and total cholesterol levels by 34%. (83) Ernst (84) drew attention to the effects of omega-3 fatty acids on blood rheology. He pointed out that with increasing doses to volunteers, among other things, blood viscosity was lowered and red cell deformability increased, possibly because the composition of the red cell membrane had been altered. Such changes would result in improved microcirculatory blood flow. An interesting aspect of clinical studies using omega-3 fatty acids is the absence of reference to studies which reported improved blood flow. An example of this citation bias is the paper by Young and Conquer (85) who discussed the use of omega-3 fatty acids in neuropsychiatric disorders such as attention deficit and hyperactivity disorder, Alzheimer's disease, schizophrenia and depression. They stated, *"Thus far, however, the benefit of supplementation (with omega-3 fatty acids) in terms of disease risk and/or aiding in symptom management, are not clear and more research is needed."* But between 1981 when the first report was published and 2005, when their paper was published, a search in PubMed revealed 58 titles relating to "Omega-3 fatty acids and blood viscosity." The English translation of the abstract of a paper in French draws attention to a potential source of confusion relating to the use of omega-3 fatty acids. (86) The author discussed the significance of alphalinolenic acid (ALA) the smallest of the omega-3 fatty acids, but he appeared to be unaware that the presence of a functional enzyme (delta-6-desaturase) was necessary to elongate ALA to EPA which is the active agent. It has been reported that in a number of chronic conditions, delta-6-desaturase is either absent or ineffective, and although ALA was provided, a lack of EPA was manifested as increased blood viscosity with poorly deformable red cells. Although Song and Zhao (87) noted that in six of seven clinical trials, *"....EPA significantly improved depressive symptoms when compared with placebo-treated populations,"* they did not discuss the basis of the improvement in symptoms.

Thus is seems reasonable to conclude that clinicians have yet to recognise that increased blood viscosity plays an important role in depressive illness, and that EPA, by lowering blood viscosity, helps to restore cerebral blood flow to normal. Such an outcome is consistent with the observation that patients who respond to any of several treatments have been shown to have improved blood flow.

> *Nancy: Fish oil is easily obtainable from health food shops, and has many benefits above and beyond its potential for alleviating depression by improving blood flow. For this reason it would seem a very safe recommendation to try out. Les would suggest that a dosage of 6 g per day would be both tolerated and beneficial.*

(e) The use of a prescription drug—pentoxifylline.

An analysis of the 2678 titles concerning the use of pentoxifylline (Ptx) shows marked differences in the way the effects of the drug were assessed, in the 20th and 21st centuries. In the 1970s there were several studies in which the major interest concerned the effects of Ptx on blood filterability and red cell deformability. In a small number of studies it was noted that the drug led to a lowering of blood viscosity as well as referring to its fibrinolytic activity. In the 1980s, there were many papers, mainly from Germany, Italy and Russia, which showed a greater interest in the blood-viscosity-lowering ability of Ptx, and in the resulting improvement in blood flow, with particular interest in cerebral blood flow. Several authors noted that a reduction in fibrinogen levels and a lowering of blood viscosity was accompanied by improved blood flow. However, it should be noted that there was a small number of studies which failed to show such benefits from Ptx therapy.

Given the amount of published information dealing with the effects of Ptx on red cell deformability, an American study (88) is of some significance as it reported that, *"Inhibition of protopod formation by pentoxifylline is associated with an increase in WBC deformability."* In order to emphasise the significance of the finding, it was noted, *"...each WBC is equivalent to approximately 700 erythrocytes in its tendency to block 5-micron channels."* This finding is consistent with the work of others which draw attention to the fact that Ptx increases the fluidity of cell membranes, indicating that the observed improvements in blood flow are the result of improved deformability of both red and white cells.

A four-year-long study of the effects of Ptx on the blood viscosity problems in both type 1 and type 2 diabetes reported that no complications of the diabetic state developed during the four years of the study. (89) Although interest in the haemorheological benefits derived from Ptx treatment continued during the 1990s, other effects were claimed. Samlaska and Winfield (90) in 1994, claimed that Ptx had a wide variety of effects, such as, *"Immunomodulation includes increased lymphocyte deformability and chemotaxis, decreased endothelial leucocyte adhesion, decreased neutrophil degranulation and release of superoxides, decreased production of monocyte-derived tumor necrosis factor, decreased leucocyte responsiveness to interleukin1 and tumor necrosis factor, inhibition of T and B lymphocyte deactivators and decreased killer activity."* What is not known is how many of these responses are a consequence of improved blood flow. However, the English translation of the abstract of a 1997 paper in Japanese (91) began, *"Pentoxifylline has been shown to have anti-inflammatory and immunomodulatory effects including the suppression of TNF-alpha production by activated macrophages."* Such reports indicate that there was a move away from the recognition of the changes in blood rheology factors and acceptance of the fact that Ptx lowered blood viscosity and increased red cell deformability. This citation bias was manifested in two ways. Firstly, by the fact that in the period 2000 to 2011, of more than 1000 abstracts, only three mentioned blood viscosity or blood filterability. Secondly, by the accumulation of several thousands of papers reporting changes in blood rheology in major health problems, which are never given clinical recognition.

But despite this controversial background, it is reasonable to propose that the blood viscosity problems which occur during depression, will respond to Ptx treatment.

> ***Nancy:*** *Pentoxifylline is a prescription drug, and because of the medical profession's failure to engage with hemorheology and its implications for treatment of a number of conditions which could be helped by improved blood flow, it is unlikely that this will be prescribed by your doctor or psychiatrist. However, this research could be pointed out to your doctor.*

(f) Ketamine as an anti-depressant.

In 1974, Hougaard et al (92) reported that 2 to 4 minutes after an intravenous injection of ketamine, measurement of blood flow by the intra-arterial 133Xe method, showed there were marked increases in regional cerebral blood flow in the fronto-temporal regions of the brains of neurologic patients. The English translation of the abstract of an article in German (93) described the effects of an infusion of 0.25mg/kg of ketamine on blood flow velocity in the basal cerebral arteries as shown by Doppler sonography in healthy volunteers. The authors reported that after the injection of ketamine,

> *"There was a significant increase in the haemodynamic parameters and in blood flow velocities." Similar findings were reported in a Swiss study (94) which concluded, "The results suggest that ketamine may significantly influence intracerebral haemodynamics via a direct drug effect rather than via a secondary effect due to changes in arterial carbon dioxide and/or mean arterial blood pressure."*

As has been noted previously, patients who responded to treatments showed improved blood flow, irrespective of the nature of the treatment; drug therapy, ECT or rTMS, so it is not surprising that ketamine-induced cerebral blood flow would be helpful in depression. Berman et al (95) reported that under randomised, double-blind conditions, *"Subjects with depression evidenced significant improvement in depressive symptoms within 72 hours after ketamine but not after placebo infusion."* Despite these demonstrations of ketamine having a direct influence on cerebral blood flow, Zarate et al (96) studied the benefits of ketamine as an N-methyl-D-aspartate antagonist, in patients with treatment resistant depression. It was noted, *"Subjects receiving ketamine showed significant improvement in depression compared with patients receiving placebo, within 110 minutes after injection, which remained significant throughout the following week."* No reference was made to those studies which had reported ketamine-related improvements in blood flow. The benefits of ketamine were reported by a Swiss group, (97) in a study of the effects of i.v. ketamine in a subject with treatment resistant major depression. The authors noted, *"The subject reported first improvements 25 minutes into the infusion and continued to describe positive effects throughout the subsequent 7 days."* Again, no reference was made to the effects of ketamine on blood flow. From about the year 2000, it seems that due to citation bias, the beneficial effects of ketamine on blood flow have been ignored and ketamine is referred to as an N-methyl-D-aspartate antagonist. An example of the consequences of this change in emphasis is a study which declared that the *"...rapid initial anti-depressant response to an intra-venous infusion of ketamine as an NMDA antagonist at 0.5mg/kg were not mediated by brain-derived neurotrophic factors."* (98) Another study which used drugs in an attempt to alter the antidepressant effects of intravenous ketamine at 0.5mg/kg as a glutamate receptor antagonist, showed that the drugs were ineffective. (99) As previous studies have shown that patients who responded to ECT had improved blood flow and that ketamine improved blood flow, it is not surprising that a combination of both treatments would be beneficial.

Okomoto et al (100) compared the effects of ketamine and propofol as anaesthetics during ECT, in patients with treatment resistant depression. Hamilton Depression Rating Scale (HDRS) scores improved earlier in the ketamine group, in association with a significantly greater decrease in HDRS scores. The authors concluded, *"The results suggested that it is possible to improve symptoms of depression earlier by using ketamine anaesthesia."* But no reference was made to the earlier reports of ketamine-induced improvements in blood flow.

While much more could be written about ketamine, it is clear that its mode of action is through its beneficial effects on blood flow, even though the mechanism remains unexplained.

Nancy: *Ketamine, like Pentoxifylline, is used in medical settings and is clearly in the 'do not try this at home' category. As with Pentoxifylline, the most you can do is hope that your doctor would be amenable to looking at this research, and considering a trial.*

SUMMARISING LES'S WORK

Nancy: Les looks on depression as a problem of blood flow. He provides the results of his literature searches which give a number of definitions of depression. He goes on to consider theories about etiology, which conclude that etiology remains inconclusive. It seems that depression involves social, psychological, and physiological processes, while the sequence remains problematic. Depression due to external events is accompanied by physiological factors, of which the observed changes in blood flow to certain parts of the brain seem to Les to be both a central feature, and one which is mostly ignored. It may also be that blood flow problems can trigger the emotional experience of depression. Whichever way it goes, addressing life issues through psychotherapy and blood flow issues through trying out some of Les recommendations makes a sensible combined approach to sorting out depression.

CONCLUSION

Now that you are armed with the tools of NLP to help you alter the patterns of thought which underlie depression, and the tools of hemorheology to help improve blood flow to the areas of the brain which are affected in depression, we hope you will be able to clear away some of the gloom and find a sunnier outlook on yourself and your life.

Recognise that the challenges are out there, and look for ways that you can take them on. Maybe you need to join others in getting better provision for pre-school child care. Maybe you need to challenge an over-critical person in your life. Maybe you need to join a group who are fighting against the type of injustice you have experienced. Or maybe you just need to give yourself the right to carry on your own life as best you can, and feel good about yourself while doing so. Look up, smile, and let the negatives slide past unnoticed. You are a good person, you have the right to be happy.

APPENDIX A:
NLP CONCEPTS - REPRESENTATIONAL SYSTEMS

(This is adapted from the author's Expert Regular Column: 'Practical NLP, Neurolinguistic Psychotherapy for the Treatment of Depression,' Part 1, *Positive Health*, Issue 174, September 2010, reproduced with the kind permission of the Editor, Dr. Sandra Goodman.)

Fundamentally, Neuro-linguistic programming (NLP) is the study of how our brain represents and processes our subjective experience. Once we understand the sequence of mental activities that are operating in a particular situation, it gives us much more ability to control what is happening. In the case of emotional difficulties, we can find new ways to process our thinking. If we are trying to improve our performance in any area, it gives us ways to do that.

If you told Richard Bandler that you were depressed, his question would never be 'why'. It would be 'how—how are you doing that?' He would be really interested in knowing the mental steps you were taking which had the result that you felt depressed. The answer would be complex, of course, but the solution might be extremely simple.

REPRESENTATIONAL SYSTEMS

PERCEIVING EXTERNALLY (^{e})	REPRESENTING INTERNALLY	
	CONSTRUCTING (^{c})	REMEMBERING (^{r})
VISUAL REPRESENTATIONAL SYSTEM (V)		
Seeing	Visualising Future	Visualising Past
AUDITORY REPRESENTATIONAL SYSTEM (A) *Words, Sounds, Music, Internal Dialogue*		
Hearing	Imagining sound	Remembering past
KINAESTHETIC REPRESENTATIONAL SYSTEM (K) *Emotions, Sensations, (External, Internal) Motor Skills*		
Feeling	Imagining feelings	Remembering feelings
OLFACTORY REPRESENTATIONAL SYSTEM (O)		
Smelling	Imagining smells	Remembering smells
GUSTATORY REPRESENTATIONAL SYSTEM (G)		
Tasting	Imagining tastes	Remembering tastes

We use our five senses to perceive our environment, and when we are thinking, we are making a series of mental 'representations' in the same five senses:

- **Seeing:** (Visual external - V^e);
- **Remembering a visual image:** (Visual remembered - V^r)

- **Imagining a future visual image:** what will the scenery be like in the new holiday place we haven't yet **visited:** (Visual constructed - V^c);

- **Auditory perception:** hearing— includes several categories— we can be listening to sounds, words, or music (A^e);

- **Remembering** (A^r) or **imagining** (A^c) **sounds, words or music**.

There is a special category of internal auditory processing with which we are all too familiar—that stream of commentary, usually critical, which goes on in our minds, which in NLP we call internal dialogue (ID)—and in common speech, talking to ourselves!

To continue with our five senses, we 'feel'. This can refer either to sensation (I feel cold) or emotion (I feel happy). This is labelled 'kinaesthetic', so we can again have categories referring to external experience (Ke), or internal remembering (Kr) or imagining (Kc). Probably when we are considering physical performance, there should be a subcategory referring to motor skills specifically. For smell and taste, we would use the words 'olfactory' (O), and 'gustatory' (G).

APPENDIX B:
NLP CONCEPTS - EYE ACCESSING CUES

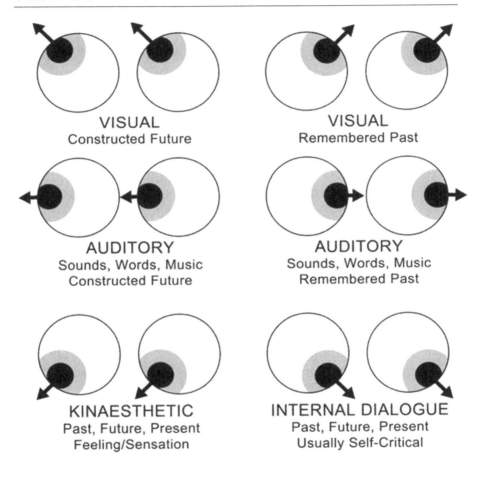

VISUAL
Constructed Future

VISUAL
Remembered Past

AUDITORY
Sounds, Words, Music
Constructed Future

AUDITORY
Sounds, Words, Music
Remembered Past

KINAESTHETIC
Past, Future, Present
Feeling/Sensation

INTERNAL DIALOGUE
Past, Future, Present
Usually Self-Critical

The direction of a person's unfocussed gaze will usually let you know the representational system in which they are processing their thinking at the time. Following a sequence of eye movements can also give information about the sequence of their thought processes.

EYE MOVEMENTS

This has been officially dismissed by researchers untrained in NLP but whose intention was to disprove its concepts. Bandler, whose philosophical position is utilitarian, would say he isn't interested in whether something is 'true'; he just wants to know whether it works.

This information has been 'proven scientifically' to be untrue (see the latest entry for NLP in Wikipedia!), and also works. If you are working with a client, using this information, check with the client whether what you are assuming is actually true for her or him. It may not be, although I haven't yet encountered an exception.

A person whose unfocused gaze, as you are looking at them, is up to their right, is probably creating a visual image. If the gaze is up to their left, the chances are they are trying to remember a visual image. You can check this, if you need to, by asking them what their front door looks like, and then what it would look like if it were painted a different colour.

A level unfocused gaze generally suggests auditory processing, left if remembering, right if constructing. (Remember the 'shifty-eyed foreigner', so beloved of Enid Blyton? If a person is thinking of what to say in another language, and then trying to remember the words for it—the eye movements will alternate—level left/level right.)

It is likely that a person gazing down to their right will be processing kinaesthetically, either feelings or sensations (again, you can check this—ask your client to let himself become very aware of the feeling of their hands in their lap, or any other sensation—and notice where the gaze goes.)

Finally, the person gazing down to their left is very likely to be engaged in internal dialogue.

Think about the severely depressed person you might see, just walking down the street. Looking down. Muttering. Now look at your depressed client, sitting curled over, looking down. Ask her how she feels and she will say "depressed". Ask her what she is saying to herself, and you can be sure her response will be self-critical. The answer to the question "how are you doing that" addressed to a depressed person, is "thinking very self-critical thoughts—and believing them—then feeling bad".

Now ask your client (or yourself, if it is you who are depressed) to sit up straight, and direct their gaze to a point near the ceiling, and try to feel depressed without letting the direction of their gaze drop. There will be a great deal of surprise when it is discovered that it isn't actually possible.

Our brain is wired in such a way that while we are looking up, processing visually, we cannot at the same time access the self-critical internal dialogue and negative feelings which are necessary to create the subjective experience we call 'depression'.

This exercise will not 'cure' depression. But learning that there is a relatively simple way to block the mental activities which characterise depression is a powerful first step in discovering that depression is not in control of you—you can be in control of it.

Your first prescription then, is to invite your client (or, if you are reading this for your own information—yourself!) to cultivate a habit (having once checked that they aren't about to trip over something) of walking around looking up—at the rooflines of houses, the tops of trees, cloud formations. Like much of NLP, this sounds so trivial as to be almost insulting, and like most of NLP, based as it is on how our brains actually process information, is surprisingly effective.

REFERENCES FOR LES' SECTIONS

1. Brakemeier EL, Normann C, Berger M. The etiopathogenesis of unipolar depression. Neurobiological and psychosocial factors. (Article in German) Bundesgesundheitsblatt Gesundheitsforschung Gesundheitsschutz 2008; 51: 379-91.

2. Vreeburg SA, Hoogendijk WJ, van Pelt J, et al. Major depressive disorder and hypothalamic-pituitary-adrenal axis activity: results from a large cohort study. Arch Gen Psychiatry 2009; 66: 617-26.

3. Scharnholz B, Lederbogen F, Feuerhack A, et al. Does night-time cortisol excretion normalise in the long-term course of depression ? Pharmacopsychiatry 2010 Feb 26 [Epub ahead of print.]

4. Piwowarska J, Wrzosek M, Radziwon-Zaleska B, et al. Serum cortisol concentration in patients with major depression after treatment with clomipramine. Pharmacol Rep 2009; 61: 604-11.

5. Hsiao FH, Yang TT, Ho RT, et al. The self-perceived symptom distress and health-related conditions associated with morning to evening diurnal cortisol patterns in outpatients with major depressive disorder. Psychoneuroendocrinology 2010; 35: 503-15.

6. Higuchi T. Major depressive disorder treatment guidelines in Japan. J Clin Psychiatry 2010; 71 Suppl E1: e05.

7. Faravelli C, Cosci F, Ciampelli M, et al. A self-controlled, naturalistic study of selective serotonin reuptake inhibitors versus tricyclic antidepressants. Psychother Psychosom 2003; 72: 95-101.

8. Geddes JR, Freemantle N, Mason J, et al. SSRIs versus other antidepressants for depressive disorder. Cochrane Database Syst Rev 2000; (2) :CD001851.

9. Geddes JR, Freemantle N, Mason J, et al. WITHDRAWN: Selective serotonin reuptake inhibitors (SSRIs) versus other antidepressants for depression. Cochrane Database Syst Rev 2007; (3) :CD001851.

10. Trivedi MH, Fava M, Wisniewski SR, et al. Medical augmentation after the failure of SSRIs for depression. N Engl J Med 2006; 354: 1243-52.

11. Herrera-Guzman I, Herrera-Abarca JE, Gudayol-Ferre E, et al. Effects of selective serotonin reuptake and dual serotonergic-noradrenergic reuptake treatments on attention and executive functions in patients with major depressive disorder. Psychiatry Res 2010 Apr 10. [Epub ahead of print.]

12. Leonard BE. Changes in the immune system in depression and dementia: causal or co-incidental effects ? Int J Dev Neurosci 2001;19: 305-12.

13. Steptoe A, Kunz-Ebrecht SR, Owen N. Lack of association between depressive symptoms and markers of immune and vascular inflammation in middle-aged men and women. Psychol Med 2003; 33: 667-74.

14. Schiepers OJ, Wichers MC, Maes M. Cytokines and major depression. Prog Neuropsychopharmacol Biol Psychiatry 2005; 29: 201-17.

15. Dunn AJ, Swiergiel AH, de Beaurepaire R. Cytokines are mediators of depression: what can we learn from animal studies ? Neurosci Biobehav Rev 2005; 29: 891- 901.

16. Marques-Deak AH, Neto FL, Dominguez WV, et al. Cytokines in women with different subtypes of major depressive disorder. J Psychiatr Res 2007; 41: 152-9.

17. Marques AH, Cizza G, Sternberg E. Brain-immune interactions and implications in psychiatric disorders. (Article in Portuguese) Rev Bras Psiquiatr 2007; 29 Suppl 1: S27-32.

18. Alexopoulos GS, Meyers BS, Young RC, et al. 'Vascular depression' hypothesis. Arch Gen Psychiatry 1997; 54: 915-22.

19. Fournier JA, Sanchez A, Quero J, et al. Myocardial infarction in men aged 40 or less: a prospective clinical-angiographic study. Clin Cardiol 1996; 19: 631-6.

20. Mathew RJ, Meyer JS, Francis DJ, et al. Cerebral blood flow in depression. Am J Psychiatry 1980; 137: 1449-56.

21. Mathew RJ, Meyer JS, Semchuk KM, et al. Regional cerebral blood flow in depression: a preliminary report. J Clin Psychiatry 1980; 41 (12 pt 2): 71-2.

22. Passero S, Nardini M, Battistini N. Regional cerebral blood flow changes following administration of antidepressant drugs. Prog Neuropsychopharmacol Biol Psychiatry 1995; 19: 627-36.

23. Bench CJ, Frackowiak RS, Dolan BI. Changes in cerebral blood flow on recovery from depression. Psychol Med 1995; 25: 247-61.

24. Cerny LC, Cook FB, Valone F. The erythrocyte in aging. Exp Geront 1977; 7: 137-42.

25. Hagstadius S, Risberg J. Regional cerebral blood flow characteristics and variations with age in resting normal subjects. Brain Cogn 1989; 10: 29-43.

26. Martin AJ, Friston KJ, Colebitch JG et al. Decreases in regional cerebral blood flow with normal aging. Cereb Blood Flow Metab 1991; 11: 684-9.

27. Alexopoulos GS. The vascular depression hypothesis: 10 years later. Biol Psychiatry 2006; 60: 1304-5.

28. Ajmani RS, Rifkind JM. Haemorheological changes during human aging. Gerontology 1998; 44: 111-20.

29. Miller SE, Roses AD, Appel SH. Scanning electron microscopy studies in muscular dystrophy. Arch Neurol 1976: 33: 172-4.

30. Simpson LO. Blood from healthy animals and humans contains nondiscocytic erythrocytes. Br J Haematol 1989; 73: 561-4.

31. Markesbery WR, Butterfield DA. A scanning electron microscope study of erythrocytes in Huntington's Disease. Biochem Biophys Res Commun 1977; 78: 560-4.

32. Simpson LO. Red cell shape in health and disease. In Swamy NVC, Megha Singh (eds) Physiological Fluid Dynamics 3, Narosa Publishing House, New Delhi, 1992, pp230-5.

33. Zucker-Franklin D, Greaves MF, Grossi CE, et al. Atlas of blood cells, Vol 1, Lea & Febiger, Philadelphia, 1981, p 52.

34. Dormandy JA. Clinical significance of blood viscosity. Ann Roy Coll Surg 1970; 47: 211-28.

35. Fishberg AM. Hypertension and nephritis. 5th edition. Lea and Febiger, Philadelphia, 1954,pp296-7.

36. Simpson LO. Chronic tiredness and idiopathic chronic fatigue – a connection ? NJ Med 1992: 89: 211-6.

37. Maes M, Dierekx R, Meltzer HY, et al. Regional cerebral blood flow in unipolar depression measured with Tc-99m-HMPAO single photon emission computed tomography: negative findings. Psychiatry Res 1993; 50: 77-88.

38. Holthoff VA, Beuthien-Baumann B, Pietrzyk U, et al. Changes in regional cerebral perfusion in depression. SPECT monitoring of response to treatment. (Article in German). Nervenarzt 1999; 70: 620-6.

39. Lucey JV, Costa DC, Adshead G, et al. Brain blood flow in anxiety disorders: OCD, panic disorder with agoraphobia and post-traumatic stress disorder. Br J Psychiatry 1997; 171: 346-50.

40. Tutus A, Kibar M, Sofuoglu S, et al. A technetium-99m hexamethylpropylene amine oxime brain single photon emission tomography study in adolescent patients with major depressive disorder. Eur J Nucl Med 1998; 25: 601-6.

41. Kowatch RA, Devous MD Sr, Harvey DC, et al. A SPECT HMPAO study of regional cerebral blood flow in depressed adolescents and normal controls. Prog Neuropsychopharmacol Biol Psychiatry 1999; 23:643-56.

42. Ishizaki J, Yamamoto H, Takahashi T, et al. Changes in regional cerebral blood flow following antidepressant treatment in late-life depression. Int J Geriatr Psychiatry 2008; 23: 805-11.

43. Ogura A, Mormobu S, Kawasatsu S, et al. Changes in regional brain activity in major depression after successful treatment with antidepressant drugs. Acta Psychiatr Scand 1998; 98: 54-9.

44. Milo TJ, Kaufman GE, Barnes WE, et al. Changes in regional cerebral blood flow after electroconvulsive therapy for depression. J ECT 2001; 17: 15-21.

45. Vangu MD, Esser JD, Boyd IH, et al. Effects of electroconvulsive therapy on regional cerebral blood flow measured by 99m technetium HMPAO SPECT. Prog Neuropsychopharmacol Biol Psychiatry 2003; 27: 15-9.

46. Navarro V, Gasto C, Lomeria F, et al. Frontal cerebral perfusion after antidepressant drug treatment versus ECT in elderly patients with major depression: a 12-month follow-up control study. J Clin Psychiatry 2004; 65: 656-61.

47. George MS, Wassermann EM, Williams WA, et al. Daily repetitive transcranial magnetic stimulation (rTMS) improves mood in depression. Neuroreport 1995; 6: 1853-6.

48. Loo C, Mitchell P, Sactdev P, et al. Double-blind controlled investigation of transcranial magnetic stimulation for the treatment of resistant major depression. Am J Psychiatry 1999; 156: 945-8.

49. McLoughlin DM, Mogg A, Eranti S, et al. The clinical effectiveness and cost of repetitive transcranial magnetic stimulation versus electroconvulsive therapy in severe depression – a multicentre pragmatic randomised controlled trial and economic analysis. Health Technol Assess 2007; 11: 1-54.

50. Speer AM, Kimbrell TA, Wassermann EM, et al. Opposite effects of high and low frequency rTMS on regional brain activity in depressed patients. Biol Psychiatry 2000; 48: 1133-41.

51. Dintenfass L. Rheology of blood in diagnostic and preventive medicine. Butterworth & Co, London, 1976, p241.

52. Rasmussen H, Lake W, Allen JE. The effect of catecholamines and prostaglandins upon human and rat erythrocytes. Biochim Biophys Acta 1975; 411: 63-73.

53. Martin AJ, Friston KJ, Colebitch JG, et al. Decreases in regional cerebral blood flow with normal aging. Cereb Blood Flow Metab 1991; 11: 684-89.

54. Carallo C, Irace C, De Franeschi MS, et al. The effect of aging on blood and plasma viscosity. Clin Hemorheol Microcirc 2011; 47: 67-74.

55. Simpson LO, O'Neill DJ. Red cell shape changes in the blood of people 60 years of age and older imply a role for blood rheology in the aging process. Gerontology 2003; 49: 310-5.

56. Simpson LO, Shand BI, Olds RJ. Blood rheology and myalgic encephalomyelitis: a pilot study. Pathology 1986; 18: 190-2.

57. Simpson LO. Nondiscocytic erythrocytes in myalgic encephalomyelitis. NZ Med J 1989; 102: 106-7.

58. Swank RL, Goodwin J. Review of MS patient survival on a Swank low saturated fat diet. Nutrition 2003; 19: 161-2.

59. Ornish D, Brown SE, Scherwitz LW, et al. Can lifestyle changes reverse coronary heart disease ? Lancet 1990; 1: 129-33.

60. Esselstyn CB, Ellis SG, Medendorp SV, et al. A strategy to arrest and reverse coronary heart disease: a 5-year longitudinal study of a single physician's practice. J Family Practice 1995; 41: 560-8.

61. French JE. Atherosclerosis. In Florey H. (Ed) General Pathology 2nd edition, Lloyd-Luke (Medical books),London, 1958, pp351-57.

62. Simpson LO. Biological thixotropy of basement membranes: the key to the understanding of capillary permeability. In Garlick D (Ed), Progress in microcirculation research, Committee in Postgraduate Medical Education, The University of New South Wales,1981,pp55-66.

63. Kaperonis AA, Michelson CB, Askanazi J, et al. Effects of total hip replacement and bed rest on blood rheology and red cell metabolism. J Trauma 1988; 28: 453-7.

64. Eichner ER. Exercise and arthritis. The haematology of inactivity. Rheum Dis Clin North Am 1990; 16: 815-25.

65. Blumenthal JA, Babyak MA, Moore KA, et al. Effects of exercise training on older patients with major depression. Arch Intern Med 1999; 159: 2349-56.

66. Babyak MA, Blumenthal JA, Herman S. Exercise treatment for major depression: maintenance of therapeutic benefit at 10 months. Psychosom Med 2000; 62: 633-8.

67. Mather AS, Rodriquez C, Guthrie ME, et al. Effects of exercise on depressive symptoms in older adults with poorly responsive depressive disorder: randomised, controlled trial. Br J Psychiatry 2002; 180: 411-5.

68. Armstrong K, Edwards H. The effectiveness of pram-walking exercise programme in reducing depressive symptomatology for post-natal women. Int J Nurs Pract 2004; 10: 177-94.

69. Ernst E. Influence of regular physical activity on blood rheology. Eur Heart J 1987 (Suppl G): 59-62.

70. Huang SY, Jeng C, Kao SC, et al. Improved haemorheological properties by Gingko biloba extract (EGb 761) in type 2 diabetes mellitus complicated with retinopathy. Clin Nutr 2004; 23: 615-21.

71. Santos RF, Galduroz JC, Barbieri A, et al. Cognitive performance, SPECT and blood viscosity in elderly non-demented people using Gingko biloba. Pharmac Psychiatry 2003; 36: 127-33.

72. Galduroz JC, Antunes HK, Santos RF. Gender and age-related variation in blood viscosity in normal volunteers: a study of the effects of Allium sativum and Gingko biloba. Phytomedicine 2007; 14: 447-51.

73. Mix JA, Crews WD Jr. An examination of the efficacy of Gingko biloba extract EGB761 on the neuropsychologic functions of cognitively intact older adults. J Alt Complement Med 2000; 6: 219-29.

74. Hemmeter U, Annen B, Bischof R, et al. Polysomnographic effects of adjuvant gingko biloba therapy in patients with major depression medicated with trimipramine. Pharmacopsychiatry 2004; 34: 50-29.

75. Horsch S, Walther C. Gingko biloba special extract EGb761 in the treatment of peripheral arterial occlusive disease (POAD) – a review based on randomised controlled studies. Int J Clin Pharmacol Ther 2004; 42: 63-72.

76. Lindaerde O, Foreland AR, Magnusson A. Can winter depression be prevented by Gingko biloba extract ? A placebo-controlled trial. Acta Psychiatr Scand 1999; 100: 62-6.

77. van Dongen MC, van Rossem E, Kessels AG, et al. The efficacy of gingko for elderly people with dementia and age-associated memory impairment: new results of a randomised clinical trial. J Am Ger Soc 2000; 48: 1183-94.

78. Kang BJ, Lee SJ, Kim MD. A placebo-controlled, double-blind trial of Gingko biloba for antidepressant-induced sexual dysfunction. Hum Psycho Pharmacol 2002; 17: 279-84.

79. Kobayashi S, Hirai A, Terano T, et al. Reduction in blood viscosity by eicosapentaenoic acid. Lancet 1981; 2: 197.

80. Terano T, Hirai A, Hamazaki T, et al. Effect of the oral administration of highly purified eicosapentaenoic acid on platelet function, blood viscosity and red cell deformability in healthy human subjects. Atherosclerosis 1983; 46: 321-31.

81. Harris WS, Connor WE, McMurray MP. The comparative reductions of the plasma lipids and lipoproteins by dietary polyunsaturated fats. Salmon oil vs vegetable oil. Metabolism 1983; 32: 179-84.

82. Woodcock BE, Smith E, Lambert WH, et al. Beneficial effect of fish oil on blood viscosity in peripheral vascular disease. Br Med J 1984; 288: 592-4.

83. Simons LA, Hickie JB, Balasubramanian S. On the effects of dietary n-3 fatty acids (MaxEPA) on plasma lipids and lipoproteins in patients with hyperlipidemia. Atherosclerosis 1988; 54: 75-88.

84. Ernst E. Effects of n-3 fatty acids on blood rheology. J Intern Med Suppl 1989; 31: 129-32.

85. Young G, Conquer J. Omega-3 fatty acids and neuropsychiatric disorders. Reprod Nutr Dev 2005; 45: 1-28.

86. Boarte JM. Omega-3 fatty acids in psychiatry. (Article in French). Med Sci (Paris) 2005; 21: 216-21.

87. Song C, Zhao S. Omega-3 fatty acid eicosapentaenoic acid. A new treatment for psychiatric and neurodegenerative diseases. A review of clinical investigations. Expert Opin Investig Drugs 2007; 16: 1627-38.

88. Chien S, Sung KL, Schmidt-Schonbein GW, et al. Rheology of leucocytes. Ann NY Acad Sci 1987; 516: 333-47.

89. Ferrari E, Fioravanti M, Patti AL, et al. Effects of long-term treatment (4 years) with pentoxifylline on haemorheological changes and vascular changes in diabetic patients. Pharmatherapeutica 1987; 5: 26-39.

90. Samlaska CP, Winfield EA. Pentoxifylline. J Am Acad Dermatol 1994; 30: 603-21.

91. Ischii D, Yamada H, Ohya S, et al. Remission induction after pentoxifylline treatment in a patient with rheumatoid arthritis. (Article in Japanese). Ryumachi 1997; 37: 810-5.

92. Hougaard K, Hansen A, Brodersen P. The effect of ketamine on cerebral blood flow in man. Anesthesiology 1974; 41: 562-7.

93. Werner C, Kochs E, Rou M, et al. Increase in blood flow velocity in the middle cerebral artery following low dose ketamine. Anesth Intensivther Notfallmed 1989; 24: 23121-5.

94. Strebel S, Kaufmann M, Maitre L, et al. Effects of ketamine on cerebral blood flow velocity in humans. Influence of pre-treatment with midzolam or esmolal. Anaesthesia 1995; 50: 223-8.

95. Berman RM, Capiello A, Anand A, et al. Antidepressive effects of ketamine in depressed patients. Biol Psychiatry 2000; 47: 351-4.

96. Zarate CA Jr, Singh JB, Carlson PJ, et al. A randomised trial of an N-methyl-D-aspartate antagonist in treatment resistant major depression. Arch Gen Psychiatry 2006; 63: 856-64.

97. Liebrenz M, Borgeat A, Leisinger R, et al. Intravenous ketamine therapy in a patient with a treatment resistant major depression. Swiss Med Wkly 2007; 137: 234-6.

98. Machado-Vieira R, Yuan P, Brutsche N, et al. Brain-derived neurotrophic factor and initial antidepressant response to an N-methyl-D-aspartate antagonist. J Clin Psychiatry 2009; 70: 1662-6.

99. Mathew SJ, Murrough JW, aan het Rot M, et al. Riluzole for relapse prevention following intravenous ketamine in treatment-resistant depression: a pilot randomised, placebo-controlled continuation trial. Int J Neuropsychopharmacol 2010; 13: 71-82.

100. Okomoto N, Nakai T, Sakamoto K, et al. Rapid antidepressant effect of ketamine anaesthesia during electroconvulsive therapy of treatment-resistant depression: comparing ketamine and propofol anaesthesia. J ECT 2010; 26: 223-7.

Lightning Source UK Ltd.
Milton Keynes UK
UKOW06f0006140716

278363UK00018B/717/P